CHINESE HERB
MEDICINE
and THERAPY

Other Keats/OHAI Titles

How to Treat Yourself • Hong-yen Hsu, Ph.D.
with Chinese Herbs

Shang Han Lun: Wellspring • ed. Hong-yen Hsu, Ph.D. and
of Chinese Medicine   William G. Peacher, M.D.

For Women Only: • Hong-yen Hsu, Ph.D. and
53 Herbal Formulas   Douglas H. Easer

AIDS and Chinese Medicine • Qingkai Zhang, M.D. and
Hong-yen Hsu, Ph.D.

CHINESE HERB MEDICINE

and THERAPY

HONG-YEN HSU, PH.D. AND
WILLIAM G. PEACHER, M.D.

Keats Publishing, Inc. ✺ New Canaan, Connecticut

Oriental Healing Arts Institute ✺ Long Beach, California

Chinese Herb Medicine and Therapy is not intended as medical advice. Its intent is solely informational and educational. Please consult a health professional should the need for one be indicated.

CHINESE HERB MEDICINE AND THERAPY

Copyright © 1982 by the Oriental Healing Arts Institute of the United States

All Rights Reserved

Keats/OHAI edition published by arrangement with the Oriental Healing Arts Institute

No part of this book may be reproduced in any form without the written consent of the publisher.

Library of Congress Cataloging-in-Publication Data

Hsü, Hung-yüan,
    Chinese herb medicine and therapy / Hong-yen Hsu and William G. Peacher.
      p.   cm.
    Originaly published: Rev. ed. Los Angeles : Oriental Healing Arts Institute of U.S.A. c1982.
    Includes bibliographical references (p. 301-302) and index.
    ISBN 0-87983-653-9
    1. Herbs—Therapeutic use. 2. Medicine, Chinese. 3. Medicine, Chinese—Formulae, receipts, prescriptions. 4. Materia medica—China. I. Peacher, William G., 1914–   . II. Title.
    [DNLM: 1. Herbs. 2. Medicine, Chinese Traditional. 3. Drugs, Chinese Herbal. QV 767 H873c 1994a]
    RM666.H33H76   1994
    615'.321'0951—dc20
    DNLM/DLC
For Library of Congress   94-40346
                                        CIP

Printed in the United States of America

Published by Keats Publishing, Inc.
27 Pine Street (Box 876)
New Canaan, Connecticut 06840-0876

Table of Contents

PREFACE

I became interested in Chinese herbs while a research fellow on the faculty of the Department of Pharmaceutical Sciences at the University of Tokyo, following my graduation from Meiji Pharmaceutical College in 1941. Since then I have published a great many articles in scientific journals in Taiwan and abroad based on research done at the Taiwan Provincial Hygienic Laboratories, the Bristol Research Institute of Taiwan, the College of Chinese Culture, the Taipei Medical College, and the Brion Research Institute of Taiwan. Meanwhile, I have intensively studied Chinese herbal therapy.

Currently, Chinese medicine is attracting more and more international interest. Unfortunately, though, available publications on Chinese medicine are either too specialized or too technical to be easily understood by the general public. In light of this, I decided to write *Chinese Herb Medicine and Therapy*. The Chinese edition was published by the Chinese Medicine Commission of the National Health Administration in August of 1973. Next came the problem of English translation. The accurate translation of Chinese medical terminology into English presented a considerable challenge. Fortunately, Dr. William G. Peacher, on numerous visits to Taiwan, edited and helped elucidate the material and through our joint efforts the first English edition was published by the Oriental Healing Arts Institute of the U.S.A. in 1975. (The Institute itself was founded to introduce the five thousand year old system of Chinese medicine to Americans. The many unfamiliar and obscure theories and terms inherent in Chinese medicine present great obstacles in translation but we at the Institute are overcoming the difficulties step by step. Our goal is to contribute to the health of English-speaking people throughout the world.)

In hopes of providing an indispensible reference to the practitioner and to the layman, this second edition makes a major departure from the first edition. The staff of the Oriental Healing Arts Institute thoroughly rewrote the introductory text and gave the entire book a new format. Nancy Hays rewrote the chapters dealing with the theoretical foundations of Chinese medicine and wrote the chapter on Chinese medicine as applied to selected problems. She also proofread the entire text and compiled the general index. Jeannine Talley revised the chapters on herbal formulas and expanded the section on herbs by incorporating more than one hundred herbs not previously included. She also compiled the appendix. Douglas Easer corrected the romanization of all the formulas and reworked the sections on pulse, abdominal, and tongue diagnosis, expanding them into chapters. An accomplished translator of Chinese into English, he also checked the text for accuracy. Judith Haueter edited and organized the entire text in order to give the work clarity and continuity. In addition, she researched new material on the herbs and devised the format for the finished edition. I am grateful to all of them for their unstinting efforts. Many thanks are also due for the hard work and revisions done by Dr. Peacher, the translations done by Messrs. Tsao-chih Hsiao and O-feng Lin, and the final arrangements for publication of the first edition made by Mr. Handel H. T. Wu. Finally, I acknowledge my deep gratitude to the Sun Ten Pharmaceutical Works Co., Ltd.; of Taiwan for donating the publishing expenses for the first edition.

Suggestions from readers are welcome to aid subsequent revisions. I would like to point out that Chapter Eleven relies heavily on *Modern Chinese Formulas* by Dr. Akira Ishihara of Yokohama Medical University and on information supplied by the Friends of Pharmacy Association and the Modern Herb Therapy Association. I am very grateful for their contributions.

With the publication of this work I find myself one step closer towards my goal: to increase the knowledge about, and the awareness of, the efficacy of Chinese herbal medicine in the Western world.

Hong-yen Hsu, Ph.D.

Chapter One

History of Chinese Medicine

In 1927 J. G. Andersson, C. L. Bohlin, and D. Black discovered the fossil remains of Peking man (*Sinanthropus pekinensis*) near Choukoutien, China. This primitive man lived around 500,000 B.C., making Chinese history technically date from then. The first written records, however, were made during the Shang dynasty (ca. 1766 - 1122 B.C.).

For the last 270 years of the Shang dynasty, the capital was located in Yin (now Honan) Province. Liu Tieh-yun found evidence of this Yin dynasty in 1889. Suffering from malaria, he bought a piece of "dragon" bone from a drug store for medicinal purposes and much to his surprise discovered words carved into the bone. Later many *chia-ku-wen* (bone carvings) were found. They verify the existence of the Yin dynasty. Archeologists have reported discovering more than 160,000 separate *chia-ku-wen*. One hundred twenty-eight so far have been definitely dated and identified, but Hu Hou-suan claimed 148 clear identifications in 1952. According to Wang Fan's "The Historical Records of the Former Chin Dynasty," *Chinese Medical History* (December 1953), 36 pieces of *chia-ku-wen* record the names of diseases but they mention only prayers for healing and make no reference to medicine.

To backtrack even further, according to earliest Chinese history, Pan Ku created China. Fourteen separate legends describe the story. In one, three kings existed in the beginning—Sky King, Earth King, and Man King. In another, three men existed original-

1

ly—Shen Nung Shih, Fu Hsi Shih, and Shui Jen Shih. Shen Nung reputedly tasted various plants so he is considered the founder of Chinese herb medicine. *Shen nung pen ts'ao ching* (Shen Nung's Book of Herbs) describes 365 Chinese herbs and is credited to Shen Nung but owes its existence to Tao Hung-ching, who wrote it as late as 450 A.D. There are no records of *Shen nung pen ts'ao ching* in the Hsia, Shang, or Chou dynasties.

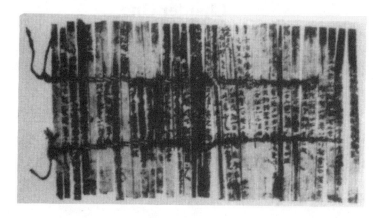

Prescriptions carved on wood strips over 2,000 years ago.

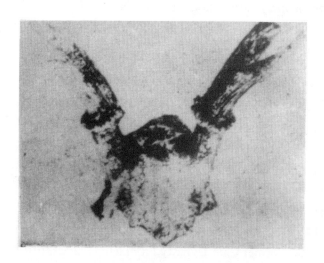 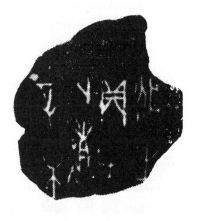

Names of diseases engraved on a deer skull more than 3,000 years ago.

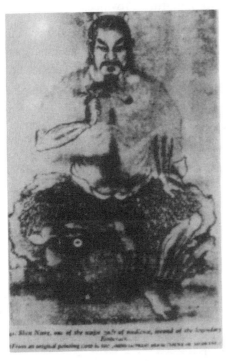

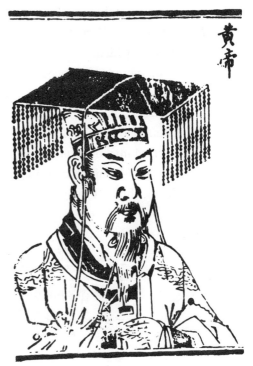

Portrait of Shen Nung (神農 , God of Husbandry, 3494 B.C.), who tasted all kinds of herbs to ascertain their healing effects. He was finally poisoned to death. (Johns Hopkins Hospital, Department of Medicine, U.S.A.)

Huang Ti (黄帝 , Yellow Emperor, about 2674 B.C.), the first emperor of China and pioneer of Chinese medical science.

The legendary *Nei ching* (The Yellow Emperor's Classic of Internal Medicine), supposedly written in the time of Huang Ti (the Yellow Emperor—2674 B.C.), records discussions between Huang Ti and six officials about the problems of medicine. Of these famous men, Ch'i Pai and Yu Fu were physicians; Lei Kung, a pharmacologist; and Tung Kung, a biologist. In reality *The Yellow Emperor's Classic* is a compilation by many scholars who used Emperor Huang Ti's name for authenticity. The work first appeared in the Han dynasty (A.D. 206). In 1835 a copy of *Nei ching tai shu* with commentary by Yang Shang-shan of the Tang dynasty was discovered at the Jen Ho Temple in Kyoto, Japan.

The original *Nei ching* consists of many parts of which the most important are the *"Su Wen"* and *"Ling Shu."* The former deals with physiology, pathology, etiology, and health maintenance; the latter, with anatomy, treatment, and the nervous system. *"Su Wen"* introduced the following methods of treatment:

    1.   *Huei shih* (cutting stone). Early surgery used stone knives and was first

performed along the Eastern coast in Shan-tung Province.

2. Medicinals. Decoctions and medicinal soups were used in Shan-si Province, Western China.

3. Acupuncture. Practiced in the plains of Southern China, Hu-pei Province, this needle therapy is widely acclaimed today.

4. Moxibustion. Heat therapy was preferred in the highlands of Northern China, Ho-pei Province. The physician burned herbs at the site of a needle inserted into the body along acupuncture meridians.

5. Massage. Manipulation and exercise were popular in the plains of Central China, Hunan Province.

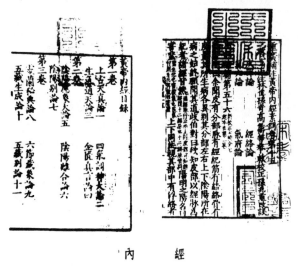

內　　　經

Nei ching (內經 , The Yellow Emperor's Classic of Internal Medicine), the first book on Chinese medical science; written 2000 years ago.

Methods for treating disease evolved gradually beginning in the Chou dynasty (1128 B.C.). During the early years, the Eastern Chou period, physicians invented and perfected acupuncture to deal with circulatory disturbances and the government set up the *Chou li tien kuan* system which divided the study and practice of medicine into dietetics, drugs, surgery, and animal care. Also, in order to avert political tragedies, an official tested all food and medicine for imperial use.

Then, during the Warring States era (403-221 B.C.), Tsou Chien proposed the Five Elements Theory which compares the human body to a small universe. The sequence of creation follows a uniform pattern: water–wood–fire–earth–metal–water. Where there is water, trees grow; friction on wood produces fire; fire turns the wood back to earth; the earth crystallized becomes metal; and metal in contact with cold forms water. The sequence of destruction or subjugation, forever ongoing with creation, follows a similar pattern: water–fire–metal–wood–earth–water. Water puts out fire; fire melts metal; metal cuts wood; wood steals nutrients from the earth; and the earth soaks up water. The theory proposes that successive creation or subjugation also occurs in the five organs of the human body. Thus the natural elements correspond to the liver, heart, spleen, lungs, and kidneys. The theory subsequently became more complicated when the concept of fate and the calendar system were added. This complication adversely influenced medical progress.

There are other sequences of "five" woven into the medical theory. The seasons and climate–wind, humidity, heat, dryness, and cold–link with the five flavors of drugs–sour, bitter, hot, salty, and sweet. The five major colors–green, red, white, black, and yellow–correspond to the five organs. For instance, yellow drugs treat diseases of the spleen and stomach; black drugs, diseases of the kidneys and bladder; and so on. If a prescribed drug is the wrong color for the affected organ, it must be dyed. The five organs also reflect a person's spiritual condition and constitute his soul and its parts. In addition, the directions of the universe are five–east, west, north, south, and center, the five directions of the wind thus influencing disease.

Myths proliferated during the Warring States era. One tells of three famous characters--Peng-lai, Fang-chang, and In-chou–seeking drugs that would give man immortality. Another, legend of the Ch'in dynasty, credits Hsu Fu with the introduction of Chinese medicine to Japan. In his search for the elixir of life, an early Ch'in emperor sent Hsu Fu with a group of children to the east. They went to Japan and never returned.

In 250 B.C. *Shan hai ching* (Book of the Mountain and the Sea) appeared. It was written in two parts, *Shan ching* (The Mountain) and *Hai ching* (The Sea). *The Sea* makes no reference to medicine but 26 chapters in *The Mountain* contain references to medicine in the discussions of minerals, animals, and plants. Examples are realgar, talcum, dragon bone, musk, *Bovis calculus, Cervi pantotrichum cornu,* cinnamon bark, angelica root, *Cnidii rhizoma,* platycodon, mulberry root bark, orange peel, jujube, *Rubiae radix,* and gambir.

During the later Han dynasty lived Chang Chung-ching (about A.D. 142-220) and Hua To (A.D. 112-212), famous and well respected physicians. Hua To, the most distinguished surgeon of his time, supposedly discovered the efficacy of hydrotherapy and medicinal baths. He also is reputed to have practiced abdominal exploratory surgery using Indian hemp (*Ma-fei-san*) as an anesthetic and to have used antiseptics and anthelmintics. Since his writings are lost, those ascribed to him are largely apocryphal, including one of the first books on acupuncture.

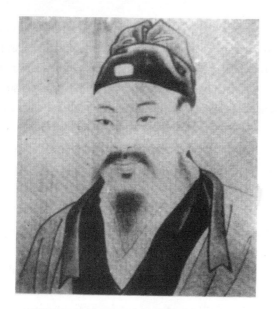

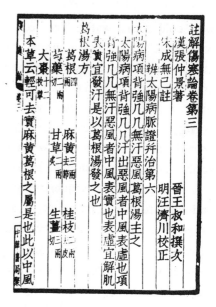

Chang Chung-ching (張仲景 , A.D. 142-220), known as "The Medical Sage", was the Hippocrates of China.

A page on Pueraria Combination as recorded in *Shang han lun* (傷寒論 , Treatise on Febrile Diseases)

Chang Chung-ching wrote the monumental works *Chin kuei yao lueh* (Summaries of Household Remedies) and *Shang han lun* (Treatise on Febrile Diseases). He discussed common diseases, the digestive system, nephrosis, rheumatism, and gynecological problems and outlined symptomatology and treatment of infectious diseases. Even more important, he separated disease into yin and yang. In *Treatise on Febrile Diseases* he categorized symptoms according to severity.

1. Greater yang: circulatory disturbances, headache, fever, chills
2. Lesser yang: a bitter taste in the mouth, thirst, dizziness, vomiting
3. Sunlight yang: weak digestion, constipation, severe fever
4. Greater yin: diarrhea, vomiting, abdominal pain
5. Lesser yin: circulatory disturbances, chills, fatigue, cold arms and legs
6. Absolute yin: thirst, absence of urination, exhaustion

In Chinese herbal medicine, disease progresses from yang through yin as it becomes more severe, and medicine is prescribed according to symptoms of yin and yang. If the wrong medicine is taken, yang disease changes to yin and the condition of the patient gradually worsens. For example, greater yang disease requires sudorifics such as Pueraria Combination; lesser yang, compromising agents such as Major Bupleurum Combination; sunlight yang, purgatives such as Major Rhubarb Combination; and yin diseases, tonics such as cnidium or *tang-kuei.*

The 287 formulas described in *Treatise on Febrile Diseases* and *Summaries of Household Remedies* and the principles on which they are based are as respected today in the practice of Chinese medicine as when they were written, and Wang Shu-ho's (A.D. 265) revision of *Treatise on Febrile Diseases* is still in use.

During the Liang dynasty (A.D. 450), Tao Hung-ching wrote *Ming i pieh lu* (Records of Famous Physicians), a revision of *Shen Nung's Book of Herbs*. It describes the classification and use of 365 herbs according to the following order:

1. Superior--120 herbs, nontoxic tonics that promote health and comfort
2. Medium--120 herbs, toxic or nontoxic, that treat mental instability
3. Inferior--125 toxic herbs that treat various diseases

Like modern medicine, drugs are divided into toxic and nontoxic.

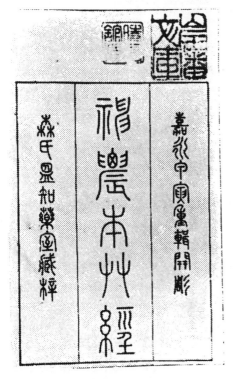

An ancient copy of *Shen Nung's Book of Herbs* (神農本草經) kept in Japan.

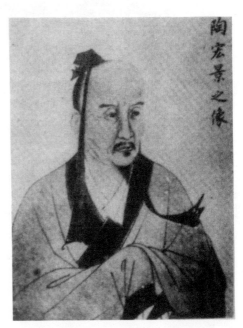

Portrait of Tao Hung-ching (陶弘景 , A.D. 425-536), who revised *Shen Nung's Book of Herbs* under the title *Ming i pieh lu* (名醫別錄 , Records of Famous Physicians).

Su Ching (A.D. 659) revised Tao Hung-ching's *Pen ts'ao* 150 years later, adding descriptions of many new herbs. The new work, *Hsin hsiu pen ts'ao* (New Revision of the Book of Herbs), covered 850 herbs. It disappeared for a long time before a copy was found in the Jen Ho Temple during the latter stage of the Japanese Chiang Ho reign. Chen Tsang-chi supplemented the *Pen ts'ao* under the title *Pen ts'ao shih i* (Supplement to the Book of Herbs) during the Tang dynasty in 739.

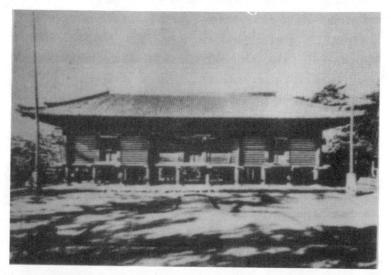

The Shosoin Treasure House in Nara, Japan, built about A.D. 756. The oldest museum in the world, it houses 56 varieties of ancient Chinese herbs.

Throughout the Chen and Sui eras (570-618), Indian philosophy and methods of treatment influenced Chinese medicine. Unfortunately, writings of this period have not survived and with them were lost many prescriptions.

In 605 the Emperor ordered Chao Yuan-fang to write a book on disease. The result, *Chu ping yuan hou lun* (On Symptoms and Causes of Disease), consists of 50 volumes with 67 divisions on 1,270 subjects. It gives the names, causes, and symptoms of diseases but no treatments.

By the time of the Tang dynasty (618-906), Chinese herb medicine had reached an advanced stage with complicated analysis and classification of disease and correspondingly complete prescriptions. Four famous men wrote medical books during this time. Sun Su-miao (also known as Sun Chen-jen) wrote *Chien chin yao fang* (Precious Prescriptions for Emergencies) and *Chien chin i fang* (Precious Supplementary Prescriptions) on medical methods of Taoism. Giving it a philosophical overtone, he prefaced his work with the words: "Life is more precious than gold." He expounded on the principles of medicine, moxibustion, and massage, and on the theory of health.

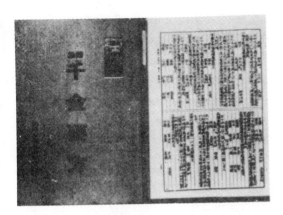
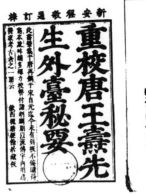
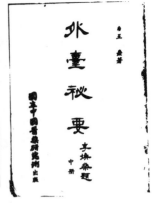

Chien chin yao fang (千金要方 , Precious Prescriptions for Emergencies) written by Sun Su-miao (A.D. 590-682).

Wai tai mi yao (外臺秘要 , Extra Medical Secrets) written by Wang Tao (王燾 , A.D. 675-755), a therapist of the eighth century.

Some prescriptions included human umbilical cord or pig and goat liver, suggesting an early form of hormonal treatment. Likewise the brain of a mad dog was prescribed for rabies, coinciding with the principles of modern immunology. Based on Chang Chung-ching's works, *Precious Supplementary Prescriptions* serves today as an important co-reference to *Treatise on Febrile Diseases*.

Three other important works came out of the Tang dynasty. First, Meng Hsien in 713 expounded on the medical value of various Chinese foods in *Shih liao pen ts'ao* (Dietetic Therapy of Herbs). Originally called *Pu yao fang* or *Pi hsiao fang* the book was renamed by Chang Ting. Next, Wang Tao in 752 wrote *Wai tai mi yao* (Extra Medical Secrets) and then in 762 Wang Ping wrote *Chi chu nei ching* (Commentary on the Yellow Emperor's Classic of Internal Medicine), the first revision of that work.

The Sung dynasty in 1010 established the Department of Medical Officials (*I kuan yuan*) and the Doctors' Clinic (*Tai i yuan*). During this time moxibustion and acupuncture gained popularity, largely because Hsu Hsi in 1034 successfully used them to treat the ailing Emperor Sung Jen-tsung. In addition, Wang Wei-i in 1026 cast a bronze man to facilitate learning acupuncture points and wrote *Yu hsueh chen chiu tu ching* (Drawings and Discussions of Acupuncture and Moxibustion Points). A great many other books of major importance were written during the Sung dynasty. The authors, subjects, or some books are listed below.

1. On pediatrics. Chien I, Tung Chi, Chen Wen-chung
2. On gynecology. Li Hsün-chih, Hsueh Chung-hsuan, Chen Tzu-ming
3. On surgery. Li Hsün-chih, Hsueh Li-chi, Chen Tzu-ming

4. On forensic medicine. *Hsi yuan lu* (Handling Grievances). Perhaps the first book dealing with malpractice and the legal problems of medicine, it discusses many research techniques.

5. *Ho chi chu fang* (Physicians' Experimental Prescriptions), compiled by Chen En-fang, includes contributions from famous contemporaries. It was revised during Emperor Sung Hui-tsung's reign by the celebrated physicians Chen Shih-wen and Pei Tsung-yuan. Such a valuable contribution to clinical medicine that it has survived to the present time, this work includes symptomatology, methods, and efficacy of herbal therapy.

6. *Fu jen liang fang* (Formulas Useful for Gynecological Problems)

7. *Ying ju lun* (Women's and Children's Problems)

8. *San yin chi i ping cheng fang* (Formulas According to Symptoms)

9. *Tai ping sheng hui fang* (Superior Health Formulas)

10. *Sheng chi tsung lu* (Catalog of Medical Formulas)

11. Concerning general health, *Pen shih fang, Tsun sheng yao chueh, Nan yang huo jen shu,* and *Cheng lei pei chi pen ts'ao*

A number of books relate specifically to drugs.

1. *Kai pao pen ts'ao* (The Book of Herbs in the Kai Pao period, A.D. 973) by Liu Han; written on order of a Sung emperor, it is a revision of the *New Revision of the Book of Herbs* with Chen Ts'ang-chi's collected principles.

2. *Jih hua tzu chu chia pen ts'ao* (The Book of Herbs of the Jih Hua Tzu School); a detailed collection of herbs, animal products, and minerals not mentioned in previous pharmacopoeias.

3. *Chia yu pu chu pen ts'ao* (Supplementary Commentary on the Book of Herbs in the Chia Yu period, A.D. 1057); based on *Kai pao pen ts'ao* with quotations of principles found in *Shih liao pen ts'ao, Shih i, Yao hsing lun* (Properties of Drugs), *Szu sheng pen ts'ao* (The Book of Dietetic Herbs), *Jih hua tzu chu chia pen ts'ao,* and so on.

4. *Tu ching pen ts'ao* (Drawings and Discussions of Herbs); an exhaustive study by Su Sung modifying *Chia yu pen ts'ao.*

During the Chin and Yuan dynasties (1211-1367), disagreement among medical authorities did much to change the practice of medicine as established during the Sung era. Liu Wan-su and Chang Tzu-ho emphasized the use of emetics, sudorifics, and purgatives, whereas Li Tung-yuan and Chu Tan-hsi used nutrients to promote and maintain health. To add to the confusion, Hua Po-jen confined his therapy to acupuncture; his principles became so widely adopted in China and Japan that the Japanese regard him as the "Father of Acupuncture."

During the Ming dynasty (1368-1643), the medical theories of the Chin and

Yuan dynasties continued to prevail. Li Shih-chen, one of the more than 700 distinguished scholars of the time, wrote one of the most famous works on herbal medicine ever assembled–*Pen ts'ao kang mu* (General Catalog of Herbs). This monumental, illustrated work describes 1,871 herbs and gives 8,160 formulas.

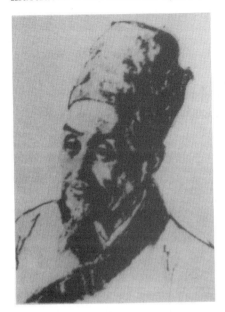

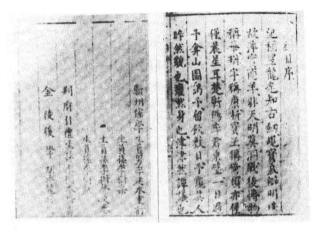

Above: The Nanking edition of *Pen ts'ao kang mu* (本草綱目 金陵本); only three copies have been preserved.
Left: Li Shih-chen (李時珍 , 1518-1593), the greatest herbalist of China.

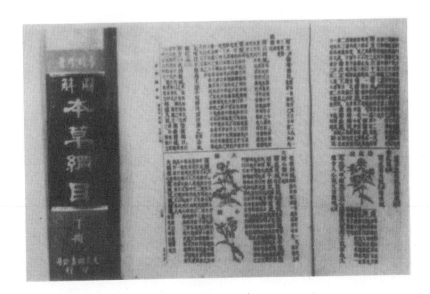

Pen ts'ao kang mu (本草綱目 , General Catalog of Herbs); contains 1,880 varieties of herbs and over 8,000 formulas.

Medical knowledge accrued during the Ming dynasty was perpetuated in the Ching dynasty (1644-1911). Unfortunately, the abundant scholarly criticism of the times did not rely on scientific principles. The better known works of this era on Chinese herbal medicine follow.

1. *Pen ts'ao kang mu shih i* (Supplement to the General Catalog of Herbs) by Chao Hsueh-min (A.D. 1765)
2. *Pen ts'ao tsung hsin* (New Edition of the Book of Herbs) by Wu I-lo; a summary of *Pen ts'ao kang mu*
3. *Pen ts'ao pei yao* (Essentials of the Book of Herbs) by Wang An
4. *Chih wu ming shih tu kao* (Plant Nomenclature and Drawings) by Wu Chi-chun

Modern Chinese herb physicians still find the second and third volumes above valuable.

Chapter Two

General Concepts of Chinese Herbal Medicine

In China and among Chinese living elsewhere, both Western and Chinese medicine are used to treat disease even though the methods and theories of the two vary considerably. The former first identifies the cause and nature of disease, then treats accordingly. The latter assesses the patient's so-called "individual conformation." The conformation is the constellation of symptoms presented–subjective and objective, physical and mental–plus the patient's general constitution and history. While Western medicine has indeed made great progress in extending human life, its treatment of chronic diseases such as hepatitis, diabetes, hypertension, allergies, and cancer falters. Interestingly, these ailments often respond to Chinese herbal therapy. Chinese drugs are made of mostly natural ingredients and as such are almost free from side effects and much less toxic than Western synthetic or natural-extract drugs. On the other hand, Western drugs, despite their effectiveness for specific problems, often produce unexpected side effects: for example, penicillin shock, thalidomide-induced deformities in fetuses, or untoward reactions to prednisolone. For this reason, Chinese herbal therapy is gaining in popularity as an alternative treatment.

Chinese medical theory basically rests upon the concept that pathways of body energy, called meridians, originate in the internal organs and transverse the surface of the body. These are the meridians of acupuncture. Before ingested herbs reach the internal organs, they pass through the meridian system, thereby producing effects far distant from the organs themselves. For example, treatment of the genitalia demands herbs for the liver, since the liver meridian flows through the genitalia. To augment herbal treatment, the meridian system may also be stimulated with massage, needles, moxibustion, ultra-sound, or laser. Meridians relate to the major arteries, nerves, and lymphatics and have many points in common with them.

Yin and Yang

Treatise on Febrile Diseases and *The Yellow Emperor's Classic* consider yang as positive and yin as negative. Yang people react to disease in an aggressive, active, progressive, and warm way. For example, if a yang person has a cold, his pulse speeds up, temperature rises, face reddens, throat becomes sore, body pain intensifies, and thirst occurs. Contrarily, yin people react to disease in a negative, passive, cool way. If a yin person—the very old and very young in particular—contracts an acute upper respiratory infection, he or she loses energy and develops a yellowish complexion and a slow, weak pulse; usually there is no fever or coughing. Although they seem healthy, yin people are resistant to cure and require extensive therapy. A Chinese doctor prescribes tonics for yin problems and sweating agents or antipyretics for yang problems.

Weak and Strong

Weak people per se lack strength; they have slack and heavy muscles, a soft pulse, little tension or tone in their organs and tissues, and a tendency to be melancholic. Strong people have tense, toned muscles; firm tissues; and a rapid pulse.

Outside and Inside

Outside refers to the external body, especially the skin. The respiratory system is also considered "outside." Inside refers to internal structures such as the digestive system, the autonomic nervous system, and the genitourinary organs.

Chinese medicine divides diseases according to outside or inside, strong or weak. The symptoms of each type follow.

1. Outside strong: tension, chills—sometimes severe, headaches, a fast pulse, and—most important—no sweating. Ma-huang Combination and Pueraria Combination are the conforming formulas.

2. Inside strong: abdominal swelling and tension, a fast pulse, yellow tongue coating, thirst. It is treated with Major Bupleurum Combination, Major Rhubarb Combination, or medications containing rhubarb and sodium sulfate.

3. Outside weak: chills, a distressing feeling of coldness, a tense pulse, head-

aches, shoulder stiffness. Cinnamon Combination, a tonic, cures these complaints.

4. Inside weak: a weak, flaccid abdomen; loss of appetite; diarrhea; abdominal swelling; nausea; weakness. Tonics such as Ginseng and Ginger Combination, Vitality Combination, or Aconite, Ginger, and Licorice Combination are the treatment of choice.

5. Outside weak, inside strong: constipation, abdominal swelling, a sinking but strong pulse. Cinnamon Combination treats outside weakness; Major Rhubarb Combination, inside strength.

6. Outside weak, inside weak: chills, fever, generalized pain, frequent diarrhea. Aconite, Ginger, and Licorice Combination treats inside weakness; Cinnamon Combination, outside weakness.

Three Yang and Three Yin–The Six Disease Stages

The major manifestation of the three yang diseases–greater, lesser, and sunlight– is sweating and fever. The three yin diseases–greater, lesser, and absolute–exhibit sweating initially but no fever because the disease is internal. The symptoms of greater yang appear first followed successively by those of lesser yang, sunlight yang, greater yin, lesser yin, and absolute yin as the illness worsens.

Symptoms of the six disease stages follow.

1. Greater yang: a mild form of disease with outside symptoms such as chills, fever, and headache

2. Lesser yang: a semi-outside and semi-inside conformation; main symptoms are chest discomfort, alternating chills and fever

3. Sunlight yang: symptoms reflect an inside problem and are more severe than greater yang–fever without chills, distended abdomen, constipation

4. Greater yin: chills, distended abdomen, occasional abdominal pain

5. Lesser yin: weak pulse, anxiety, drowsiness, diarrhea, chills, cold arms and legs

6. Absolute yin: thirst, difficult urination, physical exhaustion

The Etiology of Disease

The blood, water, and ch'i theory is the principal concept of Chinese medicine and as such has been much revised and amended over the centuries. Blood disease includes circulatory problems, including extravasated or stagnant blood; anemia; varicose veins; hardening of the arteries; and hemorrhage. Extravasated blood--an accumulation of impure blood in the capillaries, especially in the abdomen or pelvis--causes many different problems, such as generalized edema and obesity (difficult pregnancies result from the obesity), disturbances in ovarian function, a ruddy complexion, blotchy skin, an increased number of capillaries in the skin, coarse skin, and perioral bluish discoloration. With anemia, a dark violet color may appear along the edge of the tongue.

A predisposition towards extravasated blood is inherited through the mother. The condition itself may be brought on or exacerbated by injury, fever, or lack of exercise. It most often develops in women during menstruation or following child-birth. People with extravasated blood have a slow, weak pulse, show resistance and pain when the right abdomen is palpated, and are prone to hemorrhage. They are treated with formulas containing *tang-kuei* and cnidium if weak; *Persicae semen* (peach seed), *Moutan radicis cortex* (peony roots), and *Carthami flos* (carthamus) if somewhat stronger; and *Sappan lignum* (sappan wood) if vigorous. Body size also affects the choice of prescription. Large people take Persica and Rhubarb Combination; average, Cinnamon and Hoelen Formula and Rhubarb and Moutan Combination; and small or delicate, Tang-kuei and Paeonia Formula.

Water disease results from disturbances in metabolism and distribution of fluid or from abnormal lymphatic tissue and poor cellular circulation. It includes all disorders of the urinary and excretory systems. Outside symptoms are edema, arthritis, and sweating. Upper abdominal symptoms are indigestion and stomach pain; lower abdominal symptoms, frequent urination and diarrhea. Other signs are vomiting, constipation, palpitations, tinnitus, headaches, fatigue, expectoration, salivation, joint pain, asthmatic breathing, coughing, and thirst. Water diseases are the equivalent of such Western problems as gastroptosis, gastritis, asthma, bronchitis, pneumonia, pleurisy, nephrosis, and cystitis. Symptoms common to both theories of medicine include headaches, dizziness, palpitations, tinnitus, insomnia, muscle paralysis, conjunctivitis, keratitis, and inflammation of the optic nerve.

Chinese theory holds that malfunctioning kidneys cause water to accumulate in the body, resulting in water intoxication, nephritis, kidney atrophy, and uremia. Water accumulated in the stomach is called *tan-yin*; in the bronchi and lungs, *chih-yin;* in the kidneys, *i-yin*. Phlegm is concentrated water. Herbs prescribed to adjust water metabolism are hoelen, atractylodes, alisma, polyporus, akebia, ma-huang, wild ginger, and priceless vine (stephania).

Ch'i, or life energy, circulates through the body, mainly along the acupuncture meridians. *Lu shih chun chiu* (Annals by Lu Pu-wei) from the Warring States era describes *ch'i* as the determinant of life, sickness, and death in all living things. When yin and yang *ch'i* join, life begins; death occurs when they separate. *Ch'i* disease results from an imbalance or stagnation of *ch'i* in the body. Ascending *ch'i* causes vertigo and headaches and is treated with senna. Melancholic *ch'i* is treated with magnolia or perilla. Pinellia and Magnolia Combination, Atractylodes and Hoelen

Combination, and Major Rhubarb Combination promote circulation of *ch'i*. One Japanese theory suggests that an imbalance of *ch'i* causes every type of disease and divides *ch'i* into still and mobile. Still *ch'i* amasses in one place causing mental problems, such as memory loss; mobile *ch'i* flushes throughout the body causing emotional problems, such as irritability or a short temper. *Ch'i* diseases affect the nervous system, the mind, and the acupuncture meridian system. Very difficult to diagnose and cure, *ch'i* problems require the patient's complete cooperation in therapy.

Another etiology of disease is food intoxication, causing edema or auto-intoxication. The accumulation of toxins in the body results from an unbalanced diet. In young people, food intoxication develops into appendicitis, high fevers, typhoid, pneumonia, or skin diseases. Middle-aged people develop neuralgia, nephrosis, diabetes, neurasthenia, chronic constipation, and hemorrhoids. Old people manifest arteriosclerosis, cerebral hemorrhage, nephrosis, chest pain, and enlarged lymph ducts, livers, and spleens.

In all societies the medicine practiced reflects the beliefs of the people. This especially holds true in the Chinese culture because it is steeped in tradition. The seeking of the way, or *tao* as it is called, involves health practices such as following dietary laws, practicing sexual moderation, and performing meaningful work. Religion and philosophy spill over into Chinese medicine much more than they do into Western medicine, which is almost devoid of a cohesive unifying thesis. In the same vein, then, Chinese medicine is more holistic.

Diagnosis follows a set pattern based on the above concepts and philosophy. Basically doctors use what they call the "Four Diagnostic Methods"–they use their eyes, ears, nose, and hands to assess the symptoms presented by the patient. The next four chapters describe the diagnostic procedures of Chinese medicine.

Chapter Three

General Diagnosis in Chinese Herbal Medicine

Modern medicine differs from Chinese herbal medicine in both diagnosis and focus of therapy. A Western doctor diagnoses the problem and prescribes specific therapy for that problem, such as eyedrops for conjunctivitis. A Chinese herbal doctor examines the patient's entire body and situates this information within a constellation of objective and subjective symptoms–the patient's conformation. Therapy then follows according to conformation. For example, a person with a rapid pulse, stiff neck, pain radiating from the chest to the back, frequent headaches, fever, chills, and no sweating has a Pueraria conformation. He does not have this conformation if the problem is lesser yang or if his stomach is weak. People with colds, inflammation, or suppuration may be of the Pueraria conformation. Using the methods discussed in this chapter, the Chinese doctor assesses the patient's complete physical and mental make-up and determines his or her conformation.

Diagnosis in Chinese Herbal Medicine

Visual

Some symptoms are visible to the naked eye. An experienced doctor can quickly identify many problems by carefully observing the patient's appearance.

1. Physical appearance reveals general nutrition. People of muscular build with good, healthy skin are yang strong; those with the opposite characteristics, yang weak. Interestingly enough, most short men belong to the yang strong type, rarely to the yang weak type.

2. Face and skin color reveal the presence of extravasated blood and a person's general health. People with good color and clear skin demonstrate good nutrition and health and belong to the yang strong type; those with poor color and blemished skin or dry skin belong to the yang weak type.

3. Nails with a healthy pink color that quickly regain their original color after being pressed indicate strength. Pale nails that recover slowly after being pressed indicate weakness and sometimes extravasated blood.

4. Dark red lips and gums suggest extravasated blood.

5. Active, clear, expressive eyes belong to yang strong people; dull eyes, to yin strong. People who blink their eyes or shut them frequently usually are mentally unstable while those whose eyes are constantly half-shut and who have difficulty opening them suffer from neurasthenia. Reddish or violet discoloration of the eyelids indicates extravasated blood.

6. The tongue's appearance is an important aid to diagnosis, especially for acute fever or appendicitis. For example, healthy people or those with sunlight yang disease have no coating on the tongue, yet a very wet tongue without coating indicates yin disease. In general, the tongue is not coated if there is no fever. A white tongue, sticky mouth, and dry throat indicate lesser yang disease. (Tongue diagnosis is an essential part of conformation assessment. It is covered extensively in Chapter Six.)

Audient

A healthy person can differentiate among sounds, detect odors, and speak vigorously. If vocal sounds are unclear to the doctor, he suspects laryngeal, pharyngeal, or pulmonary problems of either psychological or pathological origin. Abnormal respiration also suggests problems. Gasping suggests water intoxication (pulmonary edema) in the chest; fast, short breaths are weak symptoms. Difficult respiration with shoulder movement (dyspnea) in people of delicate health indicates serious illness.

Coughing expels air suddenly and noisily from the lungs. Sputum and various accompanying sounds distinguish between types of cough and indicate the appropriate formula for treatment. For example, coughing, spasms, chest distress or discomfort, and copious liquid or sticky sputum require Minor Blue Dragon Combination; a very sticky sputum requires Minor Bupleurum Combination or Major Bupleurum Combination; and a dry cough calls for Ophiopogon Combination or Pinellia and Magnolia

Combination. Since coughs also belong to either yin or yang, formulas are likewise differentiated. Minor Bupleurum Combination or Atractylodes Combination treat a yang cough; Vitality Combination or Mahuang, and Asarum Combination, a yin cough.

Distressed gasping may indicate asthma of a degree ranging from severe to light which is further divided into inside or outside. Ma-huang Combination and Ma-huang and Apricot Combination are recommended for outside asthma and Major Rhubarb Combination and Stephania and Ginseng Combination for inside asthma. Women with a cough, suppuration, leukorrhea, and secretion require special attention.

Subjective

The Chinese doctor pays particular attention to the patient's voiced complaints in his examination. To elicit these symptoms, he questions the patient extensively.

1. Chills and a somatic cold feeling, both outside symptoms, are divided into yin and yang. A yang patient has an accompanying high pulse and fever. A yin patient has a low pulse, no fever, and fatigue. A feeling of being cold is considered less serious than chills.

2. The presence of fever in Chinese medicine is determined subjectively; it is not the objective rise in body temperature of Western medicine. People with a yang conformation always feel feverish while those of yin conformation rarely do Cinnamon Combination is recommended for outside fever; Major Rhubarb Combination, for inside fever: the site of disease is internal and severe. Alternating chills and fever, or chills with fever, are typical lesser yang symptoms. People with a severe feverish feeling are in extreme distress, fear heat or cold, and are of a sunlight yang, inside strong conformation. People who feel hot and feverish all over the entire body are of a sunlight yang conformation and purgatives are recommended. Tide fever, or a fever that comes and goes like the tide, is generally not accompanied by chills or a cold feeling. Mild fever, an inside symptom, is a low-grade fever manifested by a sensation of heat inside the body. Chest distress may be caused by fever–many people with this problem have a slight fever and should take rehmannia instead of purgatives.

3. Sweating, or its absence, helps identify disease type–yin, yang, weak, or strong. If no sweating occurs, the pulse must aid diagnosis. A weak pulse identifies the outside weak patient, while a fast pulse identifies the outside strong patient (see Chapter Four). However, outside weak also includes greater yang patients who sweat. Heavy sweating ("releading sweat") represents greater severity. A lesser yang conformation shows head and night sweating. Sunlight yang patients experience generalized sweating. If the yang patient who is not sweating continues not to sweat despite

having taken sweating agents, he may have entered a weaker stage. If so, more sweating agents are not required.

4. Appetite helps identify the stage of disease. For example, a normal appetite indicates an outside, greater yang illness while a loss of appetite with a sticky feeling and bitter taste in the mouth indicates conversion to a lesser yang illness. Yin patients feel neither hunger nor thirst but have a dry, bitter feeling in the mouth. Absolute yin patients have a hungry feeling but lack appetite and vomit after eating. These symptoms of weak digestion call for Major Six Herb Combination; no appetite and a feeling of fullness after eating call for Ginseng and Aconite Combination. Weak patients who feel full after eating may also suffer from vomiting and diarrhea or a feeling of tiredness if they wait too long to eat. An irregular eating schedule may also result in a loss of appetite. A serious condition called *hsu chung* (close to death) exhibits fever, extravasated blood, sometimes a fast pulse but good facial color, and no appetite suddenly followed by a ravenous one.

5. Thirst is a loss of saliva, a dry feeling in the mouth and throat, and a desire to wet the lips and drink water. Severe thirst belongs to one of two types, yin or yang. Yin patients crave hot liquids and yang patients crave cold liquids. Exceptions exist, however. Near the end of an illness, yin patients may desire iced drinks and severe yang patients, hot drinks. Most thirsty patients belong to the yin type and respond to nourishing herbs such as ginseng, hoelen, rehmannia, and anemarrhena and formulas such as Vitality Combination. Yang patients should take Gypsum Combination. Patients with extravasated blood may also complain of thirst.

6. Bleeding or circulatory problems require a variety of formulas, according to the other symptoms present. Warm limbs, good facial color, a strong pulse, heat, and hyperemia indicate such prescriptions as Coptis and Rhubarb Combination or Coptis and Scute Combination. Cold limbs, facial pallor, and a weak pulse suggest extravasated blood and so require rehmannia formulas like Tang-kuei and Gelatin Combination and Tang-kuei Four Combination. Tang-kuei and Gardenia Combination, a compound of Tang-kuei Four and Coptis and Scute Combination, treats both complaints. More serious bleeding (except for cases with extravasated blood) calls for Persica and Rhubarb Combination, and anemia resulting from severe bleeding calls for Major Four Herb Combination.

7. Headaches also belong to different categories, according to accompanying symptoms. A greater yang conformation exhibits a headache, fever, chills, and a high pulse. It is an external illness and calls for prescriptions containing ma-huang. A lesser yang patient has a cool forehead and a weak pulse and takes Ma-huang and Asarum Combination. Absolute yin patients suffer from severe headaches, vomiting, cold limbs, and a weak pulse—an Evodia conformation. Minor

22

Bupleurum or Major Bupleurum Combination treats dizziness, chest distress, and hardness beneath the heart. More severe distress and greater hardness beneath the heart require Pinellia Combination or Coptis and Rhubarb Combination. Patients with headaches, dizziness, weak digestion, prolapse of the stomach, palpitations, cold feet, and stiff shoulders and neck need Pinellia and Gastrodia Combination.

8. Dizziness, according to modern medicine, usually arises from disturbances in the nervous, digestive, and circulatory systems–such as anemia–or from ear or eye diseases. Chinese physicians identify water intoxication and extravasated blood as the sources of dizziness. Yang-type patients should take Atractylodes and Hoelen Combination and Hoelen Five Herb Formula and yin-type patients, Vitality Combination. Dizziness caused by extravasated blood calls for Cinnamon and Hoelen Formula in yang patients and Tang-kuei and Paeonia Formula in yin patients. In addition, yang dizziness is often attended by stiff shoulders, abdominal and chest distress, and swelling and hardness over the heart. Cardiac distress and a fluttering sensation call for Atractylodes and Hoelen Combination while a sensation of cardiac hardness calls for Coptis and Rhubarb Combination. The latter formula also relieves pain and shoulder stiffness. Yin dizziness, on the other hand, requires Vitality Combination and Tang-kuei and Paeonia Formula if in the presence of abdominal weakness, a pale face, and general weakness.

9. Tinnitus is a ringing, roaring, or hissing sound in one or both ears usually accompanied by dizziness. The three possible causes are water intoxication, extravasated blood, and food intoxication. Tinnitus caused by water intoxication calls for Atractylodes and Hoelen Combination; by extravasated blood, Persica and Rhubarb Combination and Tang-kuei and Paeonia Formula; and by food intoxication, Coptis and Rhubarb Combination and Pinellia Combination.

10. Bowel movements cannot form the sole basis for diagnosis because they fail to fall into yin or yang. For example, some yang strong patients exhibit constipation or hard stools which indicate purgatives, while others develop diarrhea. The opposite case occurs in a yin weak patient who usually has soft stools and diarrhea usually needs nourishing agents unless he exhibits constipation. People with mild constipation and a distended abdomen should be given nourishing agents rather than purgatives. Likewise, constipation, fever, and a low pulse belong to the weak category and should be treated with formulas containing rhubarb or sodium sulfate compounds, such as Aconite, Ginger, and Licorice Combination and Vitality Combination, to promote smooth bowel function. Diarrhea with palpable pain in the upper abdomen belongs to the strong category and is treated with Major Bupleurum Combination. The Major Bupleurum conformation also includes people who are aware of their own peristaltic action and develop a heavy feeling after excretion. Rhubarb or peony

23

acts as a purgative for them. However, dry stools like a rabbit's require nourishing agents, such as ginseng and rhubarb, rather than purgatives. Also included in the same category are stools of a black or dark brown color with a strong odor, stickiness, and slight moisture.

11. Urination—frequency, volume and color--fits into the yin and yang categories. The yang designation includes low urinary volume and function and the yin group, high urinary volume. The yang group further divides into weak and strong. Dark brown urine indicates yang and light colored urine, yin. Excessive urinary volume falls into a yin weak conformation. Extravasated blood with high urinary output is treated with Rehmannia Eight Formula, Minor Cinnamon and Paeonia Combination, and Ginger and Hoelen Combination as tonics. Extravasated blood with limited urinary volume calls for Rhubarb and Leech Combination. Sweating, diarrhea, and vomiting cause a loss of body fluids and hence decreased urination. Increased liquid and food intake helps to restore fluids and improve renal function. Hoelen, atractylodes, alisma, and polyporus help restore normal urinary volume. Hoelen Five Herb Formula and Capillaris Combination treat the low urinary volume and dry mouth of biliary problems.

Difficulty with bowel movements and urination are of a strong conformation. An unpleasant feeling following a bowel movement in a patient with dysuria is caused by bleeding in the urinary tract and treated accordingly. Blood in the urine caused by gonorrhea responds to Polyporus Combination.

12. Vomiting fits into either *ou ni* or *shui ni*. *Ou ni* refers to frequent retching, nausea, and dense liquid vomitus best treated by pinellia. *Shui ni* means "water vomiting," the symptoms of which are thirst and copious vomitus. It is treated by Hoelen Five Herb Formula, a compound of hoelen, atractylodes, alisma, and polyporus. Vomiting with severe headache responds to Evodia Combination.

13. Acute abdominal pain belongs to the yang conformation as do most cases of chronic abdominal pain. Hernia patients require tonics--Minor Cinnamon and Paeonia Combination, Cinnamon and Paeonia Combination, Ginseng and Ginger Combination, or Tang-kuei and Paeonia Formula. Abdominal pain in general responds to Major Bupleurum Combination, Bupleurum and Cinnamon Combination, or Rhubarb and Moutan Combination. (For further information, see Chapter Five on abdominal palpation).

14. Chest pain may be generalized or affect the ribs or the area over the heart only or be accompanied with numbness. Major Bupleurum Combination and Minor Bupleurum Combination best treat such cases. Three types of heart pain exist.

Swelling under the heart. Patients in this group complain of a feeling of distress in the chest, loss of appetite, and a sensation of softness when the chest is compressed.

They should take Coptis and Rhubarb Combination, Pinellia Combination, or Pinellia and Licorice Combination for relief.

Swelling and hardness under the heart. The doctor detects a feeling of hardness when he presses the chest firmly and the patient has a feeling of distress over the heart and a loss of appetite. Major Bupleurum Combination, Minor Bupleurum Combination, and Stephania and Ginseng Combination are recommended.

Swelling in the heart. This refers to the ascent or accumulation of *ch'i* in the chest. Cinnamon, Ginger, and *Chih-shih* Combination and Ginseng and Ginger Combination are recommended.

15. Palpitations at the lower precordium produce a throbbing sensation that may interfere with diagnosis if it spreads to the abdomen. In acutely ill people, for example, abdominal palpation seeks to detect palpitations of the underlying arteries which may be distorted by surface interference. Abnormal palpitations indicate weakness and call for rehmannia, hoelen, dragon bone, oyster shell, cinnamon, and licorice in such compounds as Baked Licorice Combination, Cinnamon and Dragon Bone Combination, Atractylodes and Hoelen Combination, and Pinellia and Magnolia Combination.

16. Swelling divides into outer and inner swelling. Outer swelling exhibits a fast pulse, sweating, and severe cold. Treatment consists of Ma-huang Combination or Minor Blue Dragon Combination. Outer swelling further divides into skin swelling and wind swelling. Water intoxication and "inside" cold cause wind swelling. Skin swelling can also result from water intoxication but is not accompanied by either fever or cold. It responds to Stephania and Hoelen Combination. Inner swelling occurs inside the body and causes a sinking pulse and difficulties in urination. It is treated by Atractylodes Combination and Cinnamon and Hoelen Formula.

In addition to the visual, audient, and subjective symptoms, a Chinese doctor notes any extraordinary odors emanating from the patient. Foul odors of the mouth or of the feces are indicative of certain conditions, much as they are in Western medicine. The finer distinctions of diagnosis lie in abdominal palpation, pulse classification, and tongue examination. The next chapters cover these important methods.

Chapter Four

Pulse Diagnosis

As a major indication of the condition of the heart, the taking of the pulse has long served as a primary diagnostic tool. *The Yellow Emperor's Classic of Internal Medicine* described the earliest method of pulse diagnosis but the detailed description has been lost. The current method utilizes the radial arteries and originally appeared in *Nan ching* (Difficult Passages) by Pien Chueh. During the Sung dynasty Wang Shu-ho made the first systematic attempt to classify pulses which he described in *Mai ching* (The Book of Pulses). He incorporated theory known at the time, including the concepts discussed in *Su wen* (Simple Questions). A paradigm divided the body into three parts known as the upper, middle, and lower warmers, each with its own pulse site.

Modern medicine recognizes the frequency, rhythm, and density of the pulse during touching diagnosis. Chinese medicine notes the following points.

1. **Pathological site.** The physician palpates the *tsun kou, kuan shang,* and *chih chung* points on the left and right wrists. According to Wang Shu-ho's theory, points on the left wrist reveal problems involving the heart and small intestine, liver and gallbladder, and kidney and bladder respectively. The same points on the right wrist reveal problems involving the lungs and large intestine, the spleen and stomach, and the metabolism and bladder respectively.

2. **Disease type.** People with a floating pulse belong to the outside conformation while those with a sunken pulse belong to the inside conformation. A floating and weak pulse identifies the outside weak conformation while a sunken and smooth pulse is inside strong.

3. **Chills and fever.** A floating and quick pulse indicates an outside fever. People with a sunken and slow pulse have an inside chill conformation while those unfortunate people with a floating and slow pulse have an outer fever and inner chills, a serious condition. Headache, fever, and chills with a floating and quick pulse indicate the outside strong fever conformation. On the other hand, headache, fever, and chills with a floating and weak pulse indicate the outside weak fever conformation. According to the great physician Chang Chung-ching, a tense pulse accompanies diarrhea and a quick, weak pulse, tuberculosis.

4. **Prognosis.** The pulse often predicts the outcome of a disease. For instance, if a person of the outside type has feelings of severe cold and a floating and quick pulse that shifts to a sunken and slow pulse, he will probably recover. On the other hand, a tense pulse in a sunlight yang patient who exhibits symptoms of irrational speech, tidal fever, and delirium foretells death.

5. **Progress of the disease.** The condition of the pulse informs the doctor of the stage of the disease. For example, a smooth, quick pulse combined with hunger and consequent overeating indicates the purgative stage. People with generalized edema, sudden stridor, palpitations, and a sunken, small, or floating pulse have progressed to an inside, weak conformation. Appendicitis with a forceful, quick pulse suggests that internal suppuration has taken place.

Pulse examination is best performed in the early morning before the patient has eaten or exercised because the pulse normally fluctuates greatly after those two activities. The physician who fails to consider this may err in his diagnosis. It is imperative that the doctor pay careful attention to accurate pulse diagnosis. If he performs the examination early in the morning before the patient has broken his fast, he will be able to detect yin (negative) and yang (positive) essences in the pulse. He should be relaxed, quiet, and free from anxiety during the examination. He places his index, middle, and ring fingers on the *tsun kou, kuan shang,* and *chih chung* points of the wrist respectively. The three points lie next to one another, extending from below and inside the ulnar prominence towards the inside elbow. His touch should be light, as if playing the piano.

Pulse Classification

		Left hand	Right hand
Tsun kou	superficial	small intestine	large intestine
(inch)	deep	heart	lungs
Kuan shang	superficial	gallbladder	stomach
(bar)	deep	liver	spleen
Chih chung	superficial	bladder	triple warmer
(cubit)	deep	kidneys	*ming men*

* Kidney function meaning the "life door." Name refers to the kidneys' reproductive and prenatal energy (*yuan ch'i*).

1. Floating Pulse

The pulse feels as if it is floating, showing little resistance even on greater pressure. This pulse is felt just under the skin with light palpation. It generally indicates an external illness and a surface yang conformation. Patients who have an acute febrile disease with a floating pulse have a surface conformation of greater yang disease. If the patient's pulse is floating and fast, it is a surface strong conformation, but if floating and feeble, a surface weak conformation. A floating and forceful pulse indicates an external firm illness. A pulse that is floating but without force evidences weakness or deficiency.

2. Submerged or Sunken Pulse

This pulse is only felt on heavy pressure and usually indicates the presence of an internal disease. A submerged and forceful pulse indicates an internal firm conformation. Patients with such a conformation should take purgatives. A sunken and weak pulse evidences internal weakness or deficiency. The presence of this pulse, besides indicating that the disease is internal, also indicates a yin conformation caused by stagnant *ch'i*. The yin conformation calls for tonics.

3. Late or Slow Pulse

A slow pulse beats less than 60 times per minute or 4 times per respiration; it generally indicates a cold illness.

A slow and weak pulse indicates weakness or deficiency and a slow but forceful pulse evidences a cold accumulation being transformed into a firm illness. The slow pulse indicates that toxins are still in the body and purgatives should be prescribed.

29

4. **Fast Pulse**

A fast pulse exceeds 90 beats per minute for adults or 6 beats per respiratory cycle, and signifies the presence of a fever in the body. A fast and forceful pulse indicates a firm hot illness while a fast and weak pulse shows a weakness or a deficient hot illness.

5. **Weak or Deficient Pulse**

This pulse feels small, sunken or submerged, and weak on light pressure. Under heavier pressure it feels hollow. A patient deficient in *ch'i* and with poor blood circulation generally exhibits this pulse picture, indicating a chronic disease with weak yang, insufficient *ch'i*, and poor circulation. Unless the pulse is extremely weak, a patient with a floating, weak pulse should be given a sweating agent. A weak pulse in a strong conformation signifies a loss of blood.

6. **Solid Pulse**

The solid pulse feels strong on either gentle or heavy pressure. It is substantial and vigorous and belongs to the firm conformation.

7. **Slippery Pulse**

This pulse feels like rolling pearls. It is observed in patients whose bodies are producing an excessive amount of mucus or who show evidence of a firm fever conformation. A slippery pulse may confirm pregnancy in a woman who has not menstruated for one to three months.

8. **Chordal Pulse**

Like the taut string of a drawn bow or of a piano, this pulse vibrates, full and long, hard and forceful--typical of many lesser yang diseases. In general, most patients with muscle paralysis or water intoxication show this type of pulse. It is also associated with abdominal pain, weak digestion, and water accumulation.

9. **Harsh Pulse**

In contrast to the slippery pulse, this pulse beats harshly, roughly, and irregularly instead of smoothly, not unlike the feeling one gets when scraping bamboo with a knife. Those suffering from a loss of blood, stagnant blood, or lack of vigor usually have this type of pulse.

10. **Tense Pulse**

When lightly pressed, the tense pulse feels like a turning rope; when pressed deeply, it feels rigid. It resembles a chordal pulse. Patients with a floating and tense pulse have a surface, greater yang conformation while patients with a sunken and tense pulse probably suffer from water intoxication.

11. Feeble Pulse

Barely detectible upon palpation, it is so subtle as to be almost nonexistent. This pulse denotes an imbalance of *ch'i*. Patients with a feeble pulse who exhibit a loss of vigor should take tonics to restore their health.

12. Large Pulse

A large pulse is forceful and full. A large and fast pulse usually belongs to the strong conformation. Patients with this pulse usually experience abdominal pain or have intestinal worms.

13. Small or Fine Pulse

In contrast to the large pulse, this pulse feels like a fine, soft thread. It is easier to detect than a feeble pulse, but it too signifies weakness. Although once in a while a strong patient has a pulse of this type, it belongs to the lesser yin conformation.

14. Hidden Pulse

In order to detect this extremely submerged pulse, the doctor has to depress the artery against the radius. Such a pulse reading indicates that the pathological site lies deep within the body. It usually denotes stagnant *ch'i* or blood clots and calls for the immediate administration of sweating or vomiting agents to expel the toxin quickly.

15. Void Pulse

Upon palpation this pulse feels broad but hollow like the end of a cut scallion. It denotes a weak conformation and is described in one of the medical classics: "Beneath the fingers it feels firm at the sides and hollow within. It is buoyant and soft." A void and weak pulse indicates that the pathological condition will soon disappear. Patients who have this type of pulse accompanied by diarrhea belong to a strong conformation.

16. Moderate

In contrast to a tense pulse, this pulse is stable, neither quick nor slow. On palpation it feels buoyant, full, and soft. A moderate pulse is a normal pulse and suggests early recovery from illness.

17. Knotty Pulse

A knotty pulse resembles a slow pulse with an irregular rhythm. It denotes an interruption in the flow of yang *ch'i* and is described in these words: "The pulse arrives slowly with occasional pauses and subsequent restorations. Such a condition reflects thriving or excessive yin."

18. Alternate Pulse

An irregular, erratic pulse beat denotes exhaustion and prostration. It is described in the medical classics as follows: "It moves, pauses, and returns. The pauses are due to exhaustion and interruption of *ch'i* in each of the five viscera." Sometimes this pulse suddenly assumes the quality of a chordal and tense pulse followed by a soft and feeble pulse. It also may become rapid and then slow, or become buoyant and then sink. Basically, though, it alternates back and forth between states.

19. Rapid Pulse

As the name implies, the pulse beats rapidly. It resembles a fast pulse but is also knotty. It alternates between being rapid and moderate. Such a condition signifies thriving yang.

20. Firm Pulse

Forceful and long upon either light or heavy palpation, this pulse does not disappear even when pressure is reduced. It denotes a firm conformation.

21. Long Pulse

In this pulse, the interval between beats stretches very long. The patient usually has an accompanying sensation of warmth indicating a pathological condition.

22. Short Pulse

In a short pulse, the beat passes quickly and feels weak. It indicates a loss of vigor.

23. Big Pulse

The big pulse resembles the large pulse but is rapid and tight. It feels like the surface of a drum: outer tension and inner emptiness.

24. Soft Pulse

This pulse, very small and soft, seems to float. It can only be felt with a light touch and indicates probable impairment of renal and/or reproductive function.

25. Scattered Pulse

This pulse confuses physicians because it feels void when lightly palpated but disappears when heavily palpated. Most patients with this pulse have a severe disorder.

26. Moving Pulse

Detected at the *kuan shang* site with the middle finger, this pulse feels very much like a pea, round and smooth. It accompanies pain.

27. Hurried Pulse

Characterized by 7 to 8 beats per respiratory cycle, it signifies a serious illness.

28. Terminal Pulses

Seven pulse types signal approaching death.

a. Swimming shrimp: just beneath the skin surface, the pulse appears and disappears. It indicates exhaustion of the large intestine

b. Pecking bird: between the tendon and the muscles; feels like the pecking of a woodpecker and indicates depletion of stomach *ch'i*

c. Rebounding stone: between the tendon and the muscles; quick and firm with a rebounding action; indicates kidney failure

d. Swaying fish: resembles the tail movement of a fish at rest; the most advanced type of an obstructed pulse; indicates uneven blood circulation, heart failure, severe chill of the three yin, and loss of yang

e. Boiling pot: bubbles like boiling soup; indicates lung exhaustion, severe fever, and loss of yin

f. Dripping rain: falls unevenly; indicates stomach exhaustion

g. Hanging rope: loose and scattered; indicates spleen failure, depletion of kidney *ch'i*, and exhaustion of *ming men*

These pulses indicating a terminal state are always uneven and scattered and usually show two or more kinds of abnormality. For example, common combinations are floating and fast, floating and late, tense and small, tense and tight, sunken and knotted, smooth and fast, feeble and small.

In sum, in traditional Chinese pulse diagnosis the pulses have twenty-eight qualities grouped into eight types according to nature and associated symptoms. The most important qualities for the physician to understand are floating, sunken, slow, and fast. Being aware of the difference in sensation between the floating and sunken qualities, the doctor can diagnose whether the surface or internal part of the body is affected. Discernment of the difference between the slow and rapid pulse enables him to know whether the illness is of a cold or hot nature. If he does not understand the differences, he may wrongly treat the illness: inside for outside or vice versa and cold for hot or vice versa. It is also well to keep in mind that in clinical treatment most patients exhibit two or more types of pulse.

Pulse palpation goes hand in hand with abdominal palpation, both falling under the diagnostic method called "touching" in traditional textbooks. The following chapter covers the intricate distinctions involved in abdominal palpation.

Chapter Five

Abdominal Palpation

Abdominal diagnosis is as important in Chinese medicine as pulse diagnosis. The purpose of abdominal palpation is to determine the presence of weakness or firmness in the patient so that the appropriate therapeutic measures can be taken. With his hands, the physician feels the patient's head, face, limbs, chest, abdomen, waist, and back to determine body temperature and the degree of moisture on the skin and to detect the presence of tumors or swelling. He also takes into account the degree of tension in the abdominal muscles. In general, if a patient's abdomen is flaccid and lacks elasticity, his vitality is weak. But if a patient's abdomen is supple and firm, his vitality is strong even though his physical condition may not be healthy.

Although abdominal diagnosis is an integral part of Chinese medicine, it has never received the attention in China that it has in Japan. In China pulse diagnosis receives greater emphasis. Abdominal diagnosis was first practiced in Japan during the Muromachi era (1467-1500). It developed into a unique system during the Tokugawa era (1603-1868). The Japanese medical authority Todo Yashimasu once said: "The abdomen is the fountainhead of life and disease. Hence, one should begin with abdominal diagnosis." Today both Chinese and Weatern medicine use abdominal diagnosis. However, Western physicians tend to note only the shape and position of the viscera.

In Chinese medical theory, the condition of the abdomen is said to reflect the internal physiological functions of the body. Therefore, the tension and strength of the muscles and the amount of pain present in the abdomen dominates evaluation of the state of the internal organs. Patients with appendicitis, for example, have resistance in the abdominal muscles induced by the muscle reflex response protecting the organ from external injury. This reflexive function of the abdomen becomes a very important index in diagnosing appendicitis; yet this meaningful pathological indication is undetectable with modern laboratory instruments.

When performing abdominal diagnosis, a physician asks the patient to lie down with legs outstretched and abdomen relaxed. (The hands should be warmed before examination.) If the doctor hears a succussion sound beneath the heart, the patient must bend his knees to relax the abdominal muscles before the examination can continue. The doctor gently touches the patient with his palms. He notes the tone and thickness of the abdominal wall and the amount of moisture on the skin and detects the presence of palpitations and swellings. Gradually a picture of the patient's internal condition emerges in the doctor's mind. The following symptoms make up the picture of abdominal diagnosis.

Clinical Interpretation of Abdominal Diagnosis

1. The Umbilicus

In abdominal diagnosis the umbilicus, considered the center of energy, is examined first. In the past, the Japanese referred to the umbilicus as "God's palace" or "God's seat." A moving umbilicus indicates weakness. People with such a condition usually have delicate health. Warm tonics such as Vitality Combination, Ginseng and Ginger Combination, and Major Four Herb Combination are appropriate formulas.

2. Thickness of the Abdominal Muscles

Patients with thick, supple abdominal muscles and thick layers of subcutaneous fat (fat which cannot be pinched together) are of a firm conformation. Major Bupleurum Combination, Bupleurum and Dragon Bone Combination, and Siler and Platycodon Formula are recommended for this condition.

Patients with thin, flaccid abdominal muscles, very little subcutaneous fat (the fat can be pinched together), cold extremeties, and a weak pulse are of a weak conformation. Vitality Combination, Ginseng and Ginger Combination, and Major Four Herb Combination treat this condition. Purgatives are contraindicated. It should be noted that patients with a flaccid abdomen and a weak constitution belong to a firm conformation if their vitality is strong. Thus, Coptis and Rhubarb Combination, a purgative, is frequently prescribed when the conformation exhibits a flaccid abdomen. However, purgatives are never given if vitality is weak.

3. Swollen Abdomen

A swollen abdomen may be present in either a firm or weak conformation. A swollen abdomen with constipation evidences a firm conformation. Peritonitis and/or intestinal colic signals a weak conformation even in the presence of constipation. Patients with a swollen abdomen and diarrhea, or a swollen abdomen due to ascites, usually belong to a weak conformation.

Patients with a resistant, swollen abdomen, constipation, and a sunken, strong pulse display the symptoms of a firm conformation. For this "strong swelling" condition, purgatives such as Major Bupleurum Combination, Major Rhubarb Combination, and Siler and Platycodon Formula are prescribed. A swollen abdomen with no resistance and a feeble pulse evidences a weak conformation, or "weak swelling." This condition needs warm tonics, such as Cinnamon and Paeonia Combination, Minor Cinnamon and Paeonia Combination, and Astragalus Combination.

4. Chest Distress and Distention

Chest distress and distention manifest a feeling of outward pressure, extending beneath the lower part of the heart at the sternum and below. Abdominal distention with resistance and pain indicates a firm conformation. A distended abdomen which is soft and not painful or resistant indicates a weak conformation. Formulas containing bupleurum alleviate chest distress.

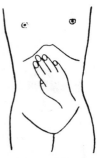

Abdominal diagnosis of chest distress and distension

a. Major Bupleurum conformation: a strong constitution and severe chest distress accompanied by constipation

b. Minor Bupleurum conformation: a weak constitution and mild chest distress with no constipation

c. Bupleurum and Chih-shih conformation: a combination of the symptoms of the previous two conformations

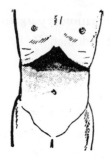

Abdominal conformation of
Major Bupleurum Combination

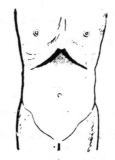

Abdominal conformation of
Minor Bupleurum Combination

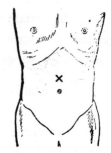

Abdominal conformation of
Bupleurum and Chih-shih
Formula

d. Bupleurum and Dragon Bone conformation: similar to the first conformation except patients have palpitations of the abdominal muscles above the umbilicus

e. Bupleurum and Cinnamon conformation: similar to the second conformation (b), but with rod-like tension in the patient's abdominal muscles

f. Bupleurum, Cinnamon, and Ginger conformation: mild chest distress, shortness of breath, and palpitations of the abdominal muscles from the umbilicus to the heart in people with delicate health and anemia

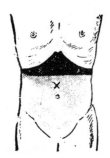

Abdominal conformation of
Bupleurum and Dragon Bone
Combination

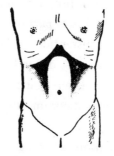

Abdominal conformation of
Bupleurum and Cinnamon
Combination

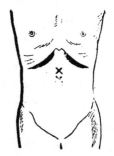

Abdominal conformation of
Bupleurum, Cinnamon, and
Ginger Combination

5. Hardness Under the Heart

A patient with stagnation and resistance in the heart area should take Pinellia Combination, Pinellia and Licorice Combination, or Coptis and Rhubarb Combination. It is a Stephania and Ginseng conformation if symptoms of asthma, shortness of breath, palpitations, edema, and hardness in the heart area exist.

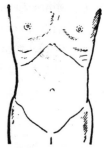

Abdominal conformation
of Pinellia Combination

6. Stagnation Under the Heart

This manifests a subjective feeling of blockage. If the stagnation lies under the heart, the physician detects a succussion sound and resistance or the patient feels pain on pressure. Weak patients are often susceptible to stagnation and Ginseng and Ginger Combination with Major Four Herb Combination is appropriate.

7. Abdominal Muscle Tension

Rod-like tension and twitching of the abdominal muscles is called "abdominal convulsion" in Chinese medicine. This condition evidences a weak conformation and should be treated with Minor Cinnamon and Paeonia Combination, Astragalus Combination, or Paeonia and Licorice Combination. Abdominal tension is treated according to location as follows.

   a. Distention and tension of the lower abdomen: abdominal distention below the umbilicus and rod-like tension of the abdominal muscles calls for Cinnamon and Paeonia Combination or Cinnamon and Rhubarb Combination. The amount of rhubarb incorporated depends upon the severity of constipation.

   b. Lower abdominal tension: tension of the abdominal muscles and the umbilicus. In Chinese medicine, the lower abdomen is known as the "lower warmer" and tension in this area is a symptom of "lower warmer" weakness or kidney deficiency. Rehmannia Eight Formula and Cinnamon and Dragon Bone Combination is the treatment of choice.

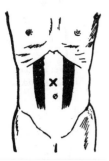

Tension of abdominal muscles

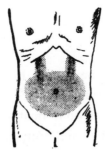

Lower abdominal distention and tension of abdominal muscles

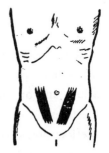

Lower abdominal tension

8. Numbness Below the Umbilicus (Weak Kidney Conformation)

A weak, empty, and fluttering feeling approximately three inches below the umbilicus typifies a kidney weakness conformation. Since no abdominal muscle tension exists, this conformation is the opposite of the lower abdominal tension conformation mentioned in (7b) even though it too identifies a weak kidney conformation. Rehmannia Eight Formula and Cinnamon and Dragon Bone Combination treat this condition. Kidney weakness, a broad term, refers to functional weakening of the lower organs. Associated symptoms are lumbago, beriberi, depleted energy, numbness of the legs, difficulty in walking, and abnormalities in urination.

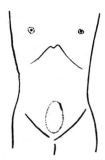

Numbness below
the umbilicus

9. Acute Lower Abdominal Stagnancy

Quick, light palpation on the left side of the lower abdomen that causes acute pain shows acute lower abdominal stagnancy. It tends to occur in women only.

10. Lower Abdominal Hardness and Congestion

A distended abdomen offering great resistance upon palpation evidences the abdominal conformation of blood stagnation. Cinnamon and Hoelen Formula or Rhubarb and Moutan Combination are the medications of choice. However, since hardness of the lower abdomen also presents when a patient is pregnant or has obstructed bowels, other symptoms should be taken into consideration before diagnosis of this disorder.

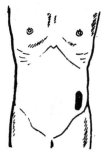

Acute lower abdominal
stagnancy

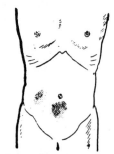

Lower abdominal
hardness and congestion

11. Abdominal Palpitations

Abdominal palpitations may be caused by poor blood circulation and/or functional disturbances of the stomach and intestines. They indicate a weak conformation for which diaphoretics, purgatives, and emetics are contraindicated. Instead herbs such as hoelen, dragon bone, oyster shell, cinnamon, and licorice are used. Among the more frequently prescribed formulas are Licorice Combination; Atractylodes and Hoelen Combination; Hoelen, Licorice, and Jujube Combination; Bupleurum and Dragon Bone Combination; Hoelen Five Herb Formula; Pinellia and Magnolia Combination; and Stephania and Ginseng Combination.

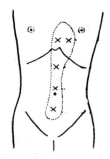

Palpitations of the
abdomen

40

12. Succussion Sound Under the Heart (Water Stagnation in the Stomach)

A splashing sound below the heart and in the abdomen when tapped lightly occurs in persons with thin and flaccid stomach walls, gastroptosis, and weak stomachs. They have water toxin and belong to the weak conformation. Formulas containing hoelen, atractylodes, alisma, ginger, and pinellia are used. Hoelen Combination, Vitality Combination, Ginseng and Ginger Combination, Major Four Herb Combination, Hoelen Five Herb Formula, Cyperus and Cardamon Combination, Pinellia and Magnolia Combination, and Pinellia and Gastrodia Combination are some examples.

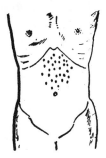

Succussion in the stomach

13. Intestinal Vermiculation

Intestinal vermiculation presents intense intestinal contractions, often accompanied by rumbling, pain, or vomiting. The afflicted's abdominal walls are flaccid and weak. However, these same symptoms may also appear with constriction of the intestinal canal, intestinal twitching, or neurosis. Vermiculation evidences a weak conformation for which purgatives are contraindicated, even when constipation exists. Major Zanthoxylum Combination, Minor Cinnamon and Paeonia Combination, Vitality Combination, and Inula and Hematite Combination are often used in treatment.

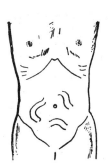

Intestinal vermiculation

14. Tension of the Central Line

The symptom of this condition is a hard, tense resistance detected by palpating the central axis that crosses 5-15 cm above and below the umbilicus. Tension above the umbilicus indicates a weak spleen which needs Vitality Combination. Tension below the umbilicus indicates a weak kidney for which Rehmannia Eight Formula and aconite formulas are frequently prescribed. Patients with acne, suppuration, and hordeolum may also have sore places along the central line that are extremely painful when pressed. According to Dr. Otsuka Keisetsu, Pueraria Combination effectively treats any of these conditions.

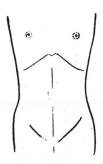

Central line tension

41

Abdominal diagnosis is learned experientially, as is pulse diagnosis. It is only after years of practice that a physician masters the art of palpation.

Chapter Six

Tongue Diagnosis

Tongue diagnosis, the last important part of Chinese medical diagnostics, dates back at least two thousand years as evidenced by the fact that it is described in detail in *The Yellow Emperor's Classic of Internal Medicine.* Chang Chung-ching's *Treatise on Febrile Diseases* also covers it and in even greater detail.

The tongue sprouts from the heart and as such is master of the five viscera and the six bowels. Moreover, various yin and yang meridians of the extremeties traverse it. Thus diseases of the circulatory system and the viscera can be readily detected by examining the tongue. It primarily reflects the presence of acute febrile and gastro-intestinal diseases.

Tongue observation helps in distinguishing between fever and chills, surface and interior conformations, and weak and firm conformations. A healthy tongue is moist and pink without any coating. In an illness that has lasted a short time, whether mild or severe, tongue diagnosis determines a chill or fever conformation. A red or yellow tongue that is thick, dry and rough, even to the point of looking charred or charred with prickles, indicates a heat disease. If the tongue is light colored or white with moist and shiny fur, or white and greasy, the disease belongs to the chill category. If the tongue fur is thin and white, as well as being slightly moist, the disease has penetrated to the interior. A swollen and light colored tongue signifies deficiency or a weak disease. A solid or firm tongue with faded color denotes severe disorders.

Chinese medicine regards the tongue and its fur as an outward manifestation of stomach vitality. For instance, in all acute, contagious illnesses or conditions involving the stomach and intestines, tongue fur often appears on the tongue. Different illnesses manifest different colors of tongue fur.

Evaluation of the tongue considers three main characteristics: general appearance, color, and the presence and color of tongue fur.

Appearance

1.   **Lean and shriveled (thin, lean, small):** a light red, lean, and shriveled tongue indicates weakness of the heart and spleen or poor circulation. If the tongue is dry and shriveled with no saliva, the disease will be difficult to cure.

2.   **Swollen:** indicates the presence of water disease toxin, excessive sputum, and flushing up of wet fever.

3.   **Rolled:** a dry, red, rolled tongue occurs with a severe fever. A white, rolled, wet tongue indicates a slight chill while a short, fat, rolled tongue accompanies moist sputum.

4.   **Projecting:** a swollen and projecting tongue is evidence of a firm conformation and indicates sputum fever in the heart. If a child is unable to retract his tongue after projecting it, his heart *ch'i* is said to be weak.

5.   **Stiff:** a rigid tongue evidences apoplexy, weak meridians, and a deficiency of stomach *ch'i*.

6.   **Protruding:** a lolling tongue denotes fever in the heart and spleen.

7.   **Tremorous:** a trembling tongue typifies "liver and wind disease." A trembling tongue accompanied by aphonia is a symptom of a weak heart and weak spleen *ch'i*.

Color

1.   **Red:** signifies a weakness of *ch'i* vitality in the heart and spleen. An accompanying feeling of surface feverishness is a sign of high fever. With weakness and internal injury, a yin weakness conformation with high fever exists.

2.   **Deep red:** indicates an incipient severe fever.

3.   **Purple:** if also swollen, alcohol toxins are affecting the heart; if dull and moist, there is an accumulation of stagnant blood. A bluish-purple and moist tongue evidences a chill toxin beginning to affect the liver and kidneys.

4.   **Blue:** indicates an insufficiency of both *ch'i* and blood.

Tongue Fur

1. **Absence of:** generally there is no fur on a healthy person's tongue. However, there is also no tongue fur present during the initial stages of febrile diseases, chronic febrile diseases, and greater yang diseases. No tongue fur on a dry tongue indicates yang disease. Gypsum Combination is used in this case. No tongue fur on a moist tongue indicates yin disease and calls for Ginseng and Ginger Combination.

2. **White fur:** if the mouth feels sticky and the throat, slightly dry, the disease has reached the lesser yang stage. The presence of extensive, thin, wet fur calls for Minor Bupleurum Combination. Thick, white fur requires Gypsum Combination.

3. **Yellow fur:** an indication of a deteriorating condition; the patient should be given Major Bupleurum Combination. However, if the tongue is yellow and wet, Major Bupleurum Combination is contraindicated. Other symptoms need to be considered.

4. **Black fur:** the result of a febrile disease. If the tongue feels hard, a purgative should be used, but if it is dry and soft, tonics should be given.

5. **Purple fur:** signifies a gastrointestinal disease.

In the following conformations the condition of the tongue takes precedence in diagnosis.

1. Stagnant blood conformation: purple spots appear around the edge of the tongue. Persica and moutan are prescribed.

2. Interior firm conformation: indicated by a short, hard, rolled tongue. The tongue shortens due to dryness and fails to uncurl after rolling. Since lack of vigor always presents in this conformation, purgatives or tonics are required depending upon the other symptoms present.

3. Yin conformation: the tongue becomes wet, thin, and black like the bristles of a hairbrush or like soot. Formulas containing aconite, such as Aconite, Ginger, and Licorice Combination, should be used.

4. Firm conformation: manifested by a red, dry tongue; usually occurs in old men who are convalescing or in women after childbirth. Treatment should incorporate herbs such as rehmannia, anemarrhena, ginseng, and ophiopogon.

Thus in diagnosis the doctor assesses the appearance, color, and fur of the tongue because its condition is an important symptom in determining the conformation.

Chapter Seven

Principles of Treatment in Chinese Herbal Medicine

Chinese herbal treatment encompasses eight methods: sweating, vomiting, purging, harmonizing, warming, removing, supplementing, and reducing.

Sweating

To expel toxins from the body the doctor induces heavy sweating. This method suits only an outside conformation–such as generalized edema, ulcers, and smallpox–except in severe cases. Two symptoms identify an outside conformation–outside chills and outside fever. In an outside chill conformation, the patient early on exhibits severe chills and fever, thirst, a white-coated but smooth tongue, headache, generalized aching, a floating and tight pulse, and no sweating or asthma. These symptoms require an acrid, warm sweating agent such as Ma-huang Combination. A person with an outside fever has a high fever, slight chills, thirst, a red tongue with a light yellowish coating, and a floating, fast pulse. These symptoms require an acrid, cool sweating agent such as Lonicera and Forsythia Formula.

Contraindications of the sweating method are severe vomiting and diarrhea, and the excessive sweating and fluid loss commonly seen during the summer.

Vomiting

The act of vomiting removes toxins from the body. Vomiting is induced only under certain circumstances, for example, when there is an accumulation of sputum in the pharynx from tonsillitis, pharyngeal paralysis (*hou feng*), or a stroke; or when there is dizziness, unconsciousness, and abdominal pain and swelling from poisoning; or when there is abdominal pain and swelling from overeating. One commonly used emetic is Melon Pedicel Formula.

Purging

Purgatives induce excretion and thus cause elimination of toxins via the colon. Cases of gastric and intestinal illness, dry stools, extravasated blood, and chronic sputum call for this method. Emetics are contraindicated. There are two types of purgatives. One type is bitter and cool, and the other, warm. Purgative drugs are either quick acting or moderate acting.

A mixed water conformation requires a water-expelling agent. The patient exhibits water distress under the heart, sweating and asthma, and a strong and solid pulse. On the other hand, a person with a hot conformation–firm sputum; pain or distress; and a smooth, solid, tense and strong pulse–should take a cool purgative, such as Lapis and Scute Formula. Extravasated blood causes abdominal swelling, increased urinary output, dark stools, and mental instability and calls for purging of the extravasated blood. Anthelmintics purge worms. Outward signs of worm infestation are heart and abdominal pain, red lips and constant hunger, and white spots on the face.

In contrast to the sweating method, purgation is contraindicated for outside conformations, semi-outside and semi-inside conformations with vomiting, or in the presence of the loss of body fluids, constipation, delicate health, or lack of vigor as is commonly seen in old age. Also purgatives must be used with extreme caution during menstruation, pregnancy, and the postpartum period.

Harmonizing

The preferred method for treatment of lesser yang diseases, harmonizing attempts to return the body to its natural homeostasis. Harmonizing serves when the sweating, vomiting, and purgative methods cannot. It is given for a semi-outside and semi-inside illness or for liver and stomach disorders.

Harmonizing is the treatment of choice for the following: (1) lesser yang diseases exhibiting intermittent fever, heart and chest distress, and nausea; (2) hot diseases, such as malaria, with thirst and nausea; (3) women with fever and abdominal swelling prior to menstruation, pain in the lower abdomen, an unpleasant feeling in the chest, and menstrual irregularities caused by liver distress.

Harmonizing is contraindicated for people with an inside or an outside illness or with a strong conformation who are suffering from thirst and impaired speech.

Warming

Warming utilizes warm and violent drugs to eliminate chills. It supplements and strengthens yang *ch'i*. Severe chills, vomiting, abdominal pain, a weak pulse, and a weak and cold conformation call for positive, warm treatment to restore lost vitality. If untreated, a loss of energy and excessive sweating or diarrhea may cause an illness to penetrate to the inner part of the body.

Chills occur in people of poor health with such problems as yang weakness of the spleen and stomach, fatigue and weakness of body and spirit, cold arms and legs, loss of appetite, stomach distress, abdominal distention, and problems with defecation.

A number of contraindications exist for the warming method. It should not be used in the presence of the following: (1) an inside fever–a deep, internal, actual fever that falsely exhibits chills on the outside; (2) a false fever inside in which there is spitting of blood and bloody stools; (3) a fever with diarrhea, hazy awareness, loss of energy, a thin and dark face, and a dry body like bleached wood; (4) yin weakness with a black tongue and dry throat.

Removing

The removing method uses cooling agents to treat all complaints of fever. The drugs employed remove heat, maintain body fluids, eliminate distress, and relieve thirst. Fever conformations divide into the essence type (*ch'i fen*), solid type (*ying fen*), and blood type (*hsieh fen*).

Essence fever symptoms are no chills; severe heat (high temperature); sweating; excessive thirst; a yellow-coated, dry tongue; and a large, fast pulse. The conformation requires treatment with acrid cool drugs. However, if the body fluids are healthy and adequate but there is fever, constipation, thirst, and a thick yellowish coating on the tongue, the bitter cold removing drugs should be employed.

A quick pulse and reddish-brown tongue characterize the solid fever conformation. This condition calls for the *ching ying* removing method.

A blood fever conformation exhibits a reddish-brown tongue, anxiety and speech disorders, mania, and spitting of blood or nosebleeds. Treatment belongs to the alkaloid, cold category.

The removing method is contraindicated for people of delicate health with visceral chills, weak digestion, soft stools, and diarrhea. Other contraindications are fever and fatigue due to excessive exercise, a weak fever due to loss of energy, or weak fever and anxiety caused by a loss of blood.

Supplementing

People with physical infirmities and general impairment of different functions need supplementation of nutrition. However, the body cannot absorb tonics in case of hypofunction of the pancreas or stomach, so the site of impairment must be considered.

Supplementation also differs according to the degree of weakness. Quick supplementation succors people suffering from extreme weakness or collapse brought on by a sudden loss of blood. Moderate tonics supplement chronic diseases requiring prolonged use of drugs. The four main conformations requiring supplementation are described below.

Supplementing *ch'i*. People with weak *ch'i* show fatigue, malaise, a disinclination to move, weakness in speaking, shallow breathing, pseudofever, sweating, a large and weak pulse, prolapse of the rectum or uterus, and hernia.

Supplementing blood. A weak blood conformation exhibits a yellowish complexion, pale lips and nails, tinnitus, excessive stomach acid, palpitations in the chest, and, if in a woman, menstrual disorders with thin and/or stagnant blood.

Supplementing yin. Signs of a yin weak conformation are slenderness, weakness, thirst, coarse skin, tinnitus, dizziness, excessive palpitations, eclampsia, insomnia, night sweats, nocturnal emissions, coughing, and spitting of blood.

Supplementing yang. Many symptoms identify a yang weak conformation: chills in the lower body, pain at knees and waist, weakness and numbness of the feet, difficulty in walking, lower abdominal pain, problems with defecation, frequent but sparse urination, impotence, and asthma.

Reducing

Hard substances due to occluded *ch'i*, blood, or sputum may accumulate and swell in the abdomen. The reduction method, resembling purgation, breaks up and disperses such accumulations. Purgatives alleviate dry stools, extravasated blood, chronic sputum, and acute strong complaints whereas reducing agents treat generalized chronic abdominal swelling or ulcers. The illness disappears only gradually because reducing agents act slowly.

Symptoms requiring this method divide into two groups as follows.

1.   Ulcers, swelling, abdominal distress, extravasated blood, fetid breath, and swelling of the abdomen or stomach. These require agents to aid digestion, that is, reducing agents such as menthol granules.

2.   Stagnant water in the stomach, hardness under the heart, overflowing water vapor, weak pulmonary function, dropsical swelling of the whole body, quickened breathing, and swelling under the waist. These require relief of water distress.

Contraindications for the reducing method are weak *ch'i* with abdominal distention; yin weak fever, thirst, loss of appetite, lowered splenic function, abdominal swelling, diarrhea, and weak digestion; weakness of the spleen and stomach with excessive sputum; and gynecological problems--loss of blood and amenorrhea.

Sometimes conformations require treatment with two methods. For instance, sputum disease, or congestion, requires a combination of methods. Following are examples of treatment using two methods.

Sweating and purging. Sweating treats outside disease while purging treats inside disease. When both conformations appear simultaneously, the outside illness must be relieved first. The inside illness should not be treated until afterwards. If both are acute, a combined method serves best. For example, severe chills, fever, and headache identify the outside conformation while abdominal swelling identifies the inside conformation. First Cinnamon Combination is given to relieve the outside symptoms, followed by rhubarb for the inside symptoms.

Warming and removing. Singularly these two methods differ as to target, but sometimes patients show complicated symptoms of upper or lower chills or fever following infectious diseases. In other cases, they undergo radical changes in yin or yang *ch'i* or in a weak or strong conformation or vice versa. Because of these changes, the use of only one method worsens the symptoms, but a combination of two secures favorable results.

Attacking and supplementing. Attacking, or aggressive methods of treatment, are purging and inducing vomiting. Only people with strong conformations require either one. Contrarily, people with weak conformations require supplements. The problem arises when a person's original strength has been dissipated fighting an illness improperly treated. As the disease roots itself more deeply inside the body, the patient develops a weak conformation. In such cases, the supplementing method would cause the illness to stagnate in one place but the attacking method would result in prostration. Thus neither method can be advised alone–they must be used together. An example would be the use of ginseng and cnidium as tonics and rhubarb and sodium sulfate as purgatives.

Reducing and supplementing. A weak pancreas and stomach or poor digestion–accumulated food, gastric swelling, shallow breathing, and loss of appetite–respond well to these methods in combination. The components of Chih-shih and Magnolia Formula illustrate this combination. Ginseng and peony serve as tonics for the spleen and stomach and *chih-shih* and magnolia reduce swelling and distress.

Principles of Treatment

Chinese medicine traditionally both supplements and purges according to the following guidelines.

1.   Always supplement weakness, if present, before purging. For example, if a slightly weak conformation mixes with a strong conformation, the weakness should be supplemented first. An inside strong conformation–constipation, abdominal swelling, thirst, bloody urine, outside chills, and weak symptoms--calls for supplementation until the chills disappear. So also, treatment of the outside strong chill conformation must follow treatment of the inside weak conformation characterized by frequent diarrhea, a weak pulse, cold arms and legs, and a headache.

2.   Treat an outside conformation before treating extravasated blood.

3.   With greater yang or sunlight yang disease, treat the outside conformation first unless the inside conformation is serious and worsening. In such a case, the order of treatment is reversed.

4.   Some formulas, such as Cinnamon and Ginseng Combination, treat both outside and inside conformation at the same time.

If the physician cannot tell from the symptoms whether the conformation is weak or strong, he should behave as if it were weak so as not to aggravate the illness–illness worsens if a weak conformation is mistakenly treated as a strong one.

If a patient under treatment for a chronic problem suddenly develops an acute illness, the physician should suspend therapy for the former and immediately treat the latter. For example, a patient with gallstones who develops an upper respiratory infection should stop taking formulas for gallstones and start ones for the new problem.

Sometimes medication takes two to three days to produce noticeable improvement. If improvement occurs, the patient should obviously continue taking that formula. Not so obvious, however, is the necessity to continue the formula if no changes or negative changes (*ming husan*) occur. Sometimes after a turn for the worse, however, the sickness becomes more amenable to treatment. For example, a patient taking Pinellia and Ginger Combination will usually suddenly vomit a large quantity of water and soon find his stomach disease cured. The same change for the better may follow uterine bleeding in an asthma patient taking Minor Blue Dragon Combination. Despite evident negative side effects, the medicine has done its job.

Chapter Eight

Chinese Medical Theory on Selected Problems

Chinese herbal medicine as practiced today incorporates a great deal of Western medical theory. However, a uniquely Chinese approach exists for certain problems because of the Chinese physician's reliance on conformation in diagnosis. For example, *ch'i* or blood disease matches no specific Western diagnosis. They are unique to Chinese medicine. Such problems as hypertension or rheumatism, on the other hand, are known to physicians of both cultures even though the theory underlying the cause and therapy differ widely. The purpose of this chapter is to explore those medical problems which Chinese medicine approaches independently of Western theory.

Two examples illustrate the uniqueness of Chinese theory: pain and stagnant blood. The underlying causes of pain are many, ranging from chills to fever to obstructed *ch'i*, yet only one cause–stagnant blood–brings on all gynecological pain. For this reason gynecological problems, although common and varied, are not treated as separate ailments because they all have only one cause–stagnant blood or blood disease.

Blood Disease

Impaired circulation of blood causes stagnation and extravasation. It most often occurs in women during menopause or after surgery because of increased resistance of the liver capillaries, poor splenic function, and accumulation of heat in the liver. Stagnant blood generates a great many symptoms. They include lower abdominal pain, sexual dysfunction, malaise, emotional instability, dizziness, heaviness in the head, poor memory, dark circles under the eyes, rough skin, dark lips, a dark violet tongue, shoulder stiffness, cold legs and feet, black feces, and a dry mouth with an inability to drink. Women with stagnant blood suffer from irregular menstruation, leukorrhea, and endometriosis.

The other common blood disease is weakness of the blood, or anemia. The conformation presents pallor, a pale red tongue, irritability, insomnia, palpitations, nocturnal fever, night sweats, and pale nail beds.

Ch'i Disease

Chapter Two presented the basic theory of *ch'i*, one of the three humors. External injury, dietary imbalance, or emotional distress interferes with the proper circulation of *ch'i*. If *ch'i* flows in a direction opposite to its natural course along the meridians, resultant symptoms might be palpitations, headaches, hysteria, emotional instability, rushing of blood to the head, dizziness, a cold lower abdomen, and sensations of energy rushing from the abdomen to the heart. On the other hand, stagnated or obstructed *ch'i* produces the sensation of a lump in the throat or a heavy feeling in the abdomen often accompanied by nervous symptoms. Weak *ch'i* exhibits shortness of breath; sweating; vertigo; palpitations; a disinclination to talk; a moist, white tongue; and a sunken, slow, feeble pulse.

Water Accumulation

Imbalances in water metabolism result in accumulation of fluids (see Chapter Two). Water pooling in skin tissue gives rise to rheumatic problems; in the stomach, atony and distention and prolapse; in the lungs and heart, coughing and chest pain with dyspnea; in the kidneys, edema and nephritis; in the brain, dizziness and headaches. Stagnant water beneath the heart causes pain on the same level in the back.

Hidden water may cause an incredible variety of seemingly unrelated symptoms. Some of the possibilities are asthma, tinnitus, insomnia, constipation, vomiting, joint pain, obesity, mental illness, eczema, and bladder infections.

The major formula for all water diseases is Hoelen Five Herb Formula, a diuretic.

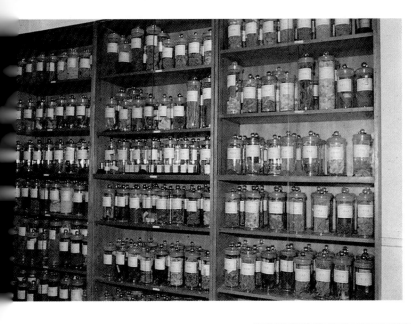

Specimens
of Chinese herb drugs

Microscopic examination
of a Chinese herb

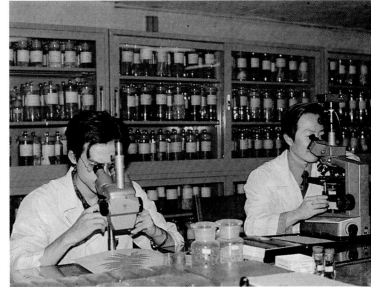

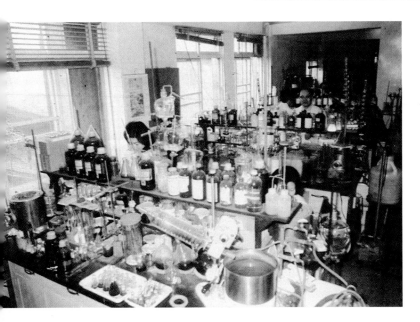

Laboratory for
studying Chinese herbs

Some modern equipment used for identifying and assaying Chinese herb drugs

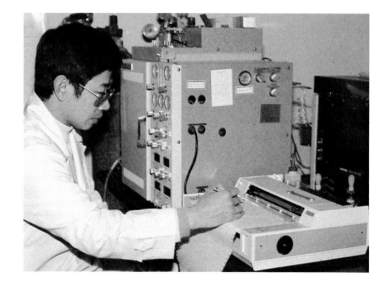

Gas chromatograph

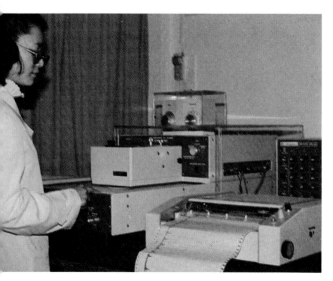

Dual wavelength TLC scanner

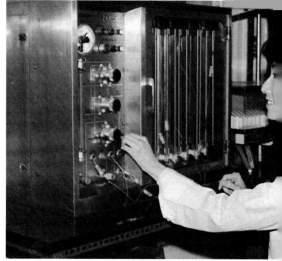

Droplet countercurrent chromatograph

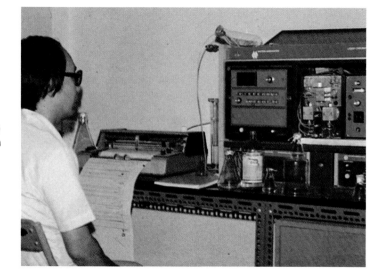

High performance
liquid chromatograph

Pharmacologic tests of herb activity

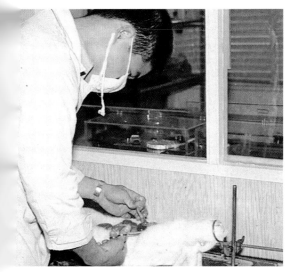

Animal test

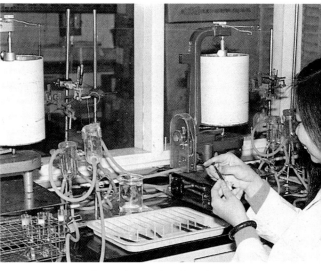

Smooth muscle relaxation test

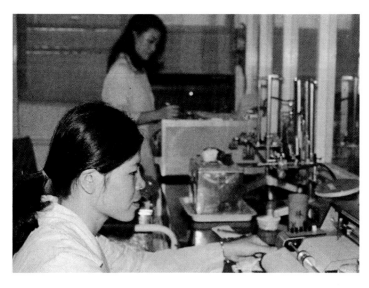

Platelet coagulation test and hypotension test

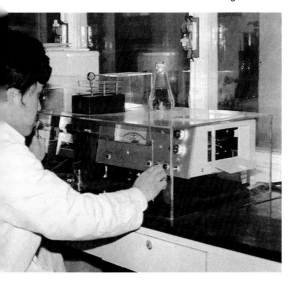

Flame photometer for diuresis test

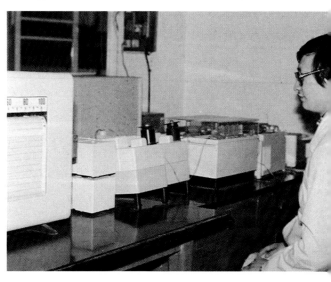

Hypoglycemic and hypocholesterolemic tests

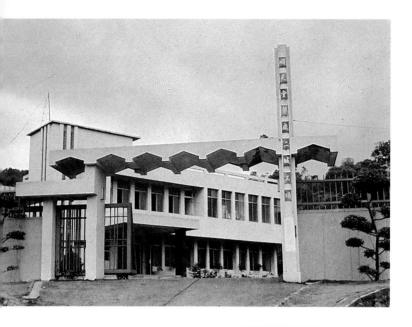

Sun Ten Pharmaceutical
Works Co., Ltd.
a modernized Chinese
drug manufactory

Extraction equipment

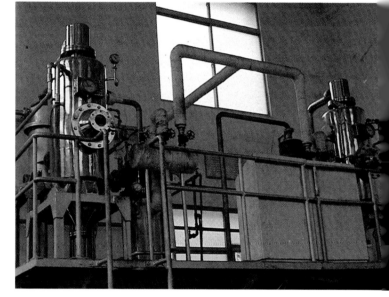

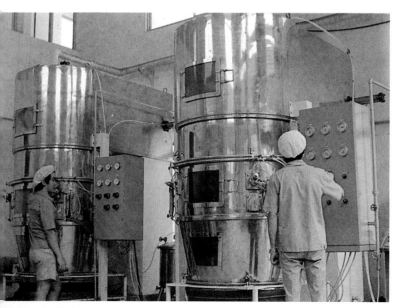

High-vacuum
spray-drying equipment

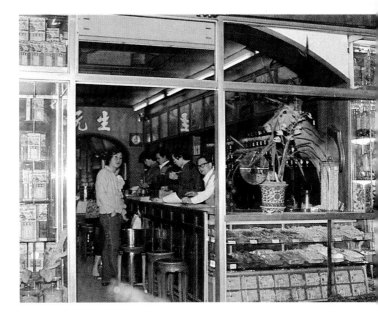

Front view of a Chinese
drug store in Taipei

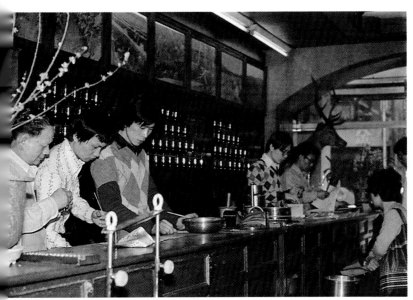

Dispensing at a Chinese
drug store in Taipei

Drs. William G. Peacher and
Hong-Yen Hsu at a modern
Chinese drug store

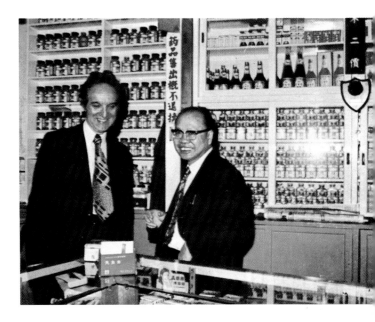

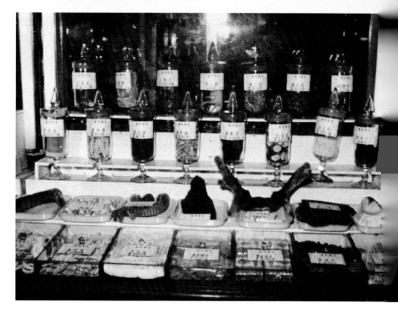

Some precious Chinese herbs
displayed at a Chinese drug
store in Taipei

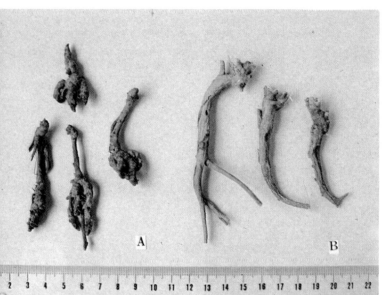

A: Coptidis Rhizoma
B: Bupleuri Radix

A: Angelicae Radix
B: Glycyrrhizae Radix
C: Cinnamomi Cortex

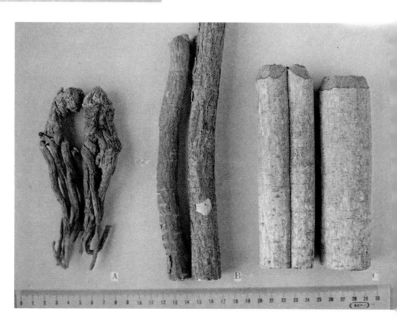

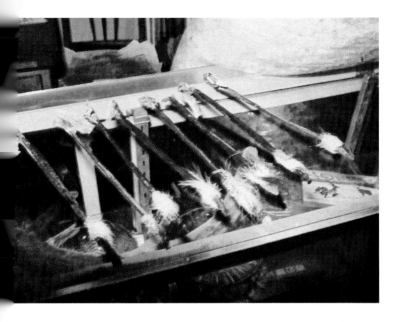

Penis et Testis Cervi
displayed at a Chinese
drug store

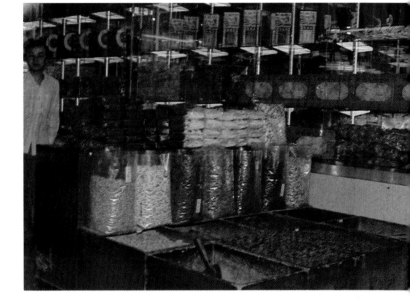

Some edible Chinese herbs

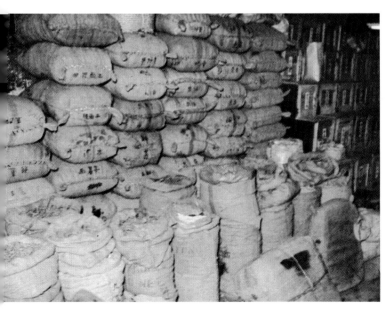

A wholesale Chinese drug
dealer in Taipei

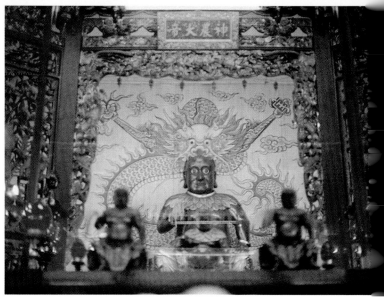

God of Husbandry,
Shen Nung, the god of
Chinese medicine

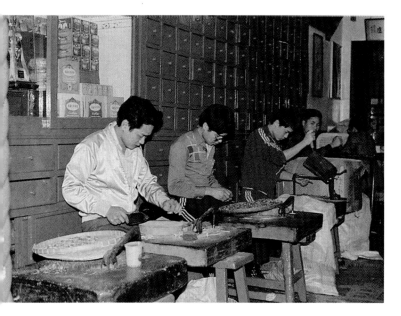

Processing Chinese herbs

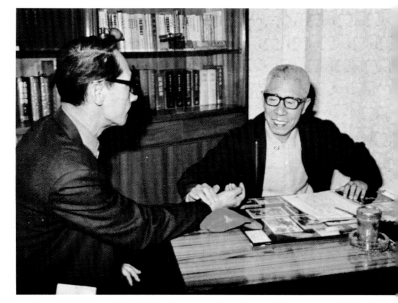

Pulse palpation by a
Chinese herb doctor

Pain

Somatic Pain

Somatic pain means the whole body aches and hurts. It differs from chronic, recurrent attacks of pain followed by numbness. Somatic pain resulting from infection requires dispersing formulas for alleviation. That induced by internal injury results from deficient *ch'i,* blood, or yin. Somatic pain is classified according to cause. The following describe the many types of conformations involving somatic pain.

1. Chills from external toxins (influenza). Symptoms are severe chills, no sweating, a stuffy nose and sniffling, somatic aches and pain, and a floating, tight pulse.

2. Malnourishment. If the patient aches all over and has a sunken, late pulse after sweating, it is because the flow of yin has been impaired by sweating and malnourishment. Muscle atrophy results.

3. Accumulation of wet toxin. Wet toxin adhering to the muscles causes somatic pain. The patient may even have trouble turning his body. Treatment utilizes anti-wet formulas.

4. Fever of the heart and lungs. This lukewarm disease exhibits fever, sweating with no reduction of fever, snoring, lethargy, a feeling of heaviness, and somatic pain.

5. Descending yang. Excessive hunger, overeating, or overwork may lead the flow of yang to descend causing heaviness of the limbs and somatic pain.

6. Agitated depression. Weakness of the blood and melancholic heat cause sudden chills and fever during menstruation or after childbirth, accompanied with chest distention, irritability, and somatic pain.

Shoulder and Back Pain

Shoulder and back pain result either from infection or internal injury. Acute pain indicates an infection while chronic aching indicates an internal injury.

1. Cold pain induced by infection. Chills induced by infection impair circulation along the greater yang bladder meridian of the feet (extending from neck to ankle) and cause a stiff neck, severe chills, absence of sweating, and a floating, tight pulse.

2. Phlegm. When congestion attacks the shoulder and back meridian, it prevents proper blood circulation; possible ensuing symptoms are stagnant liquid in the stomach, pain in the shoulders and back, and aching, weak hands and arms. Expectorants prove effective for such cases. Patients may also experience chills in the shoulders and back or chills and pain in either the stomach or the area of the back opposite the stomach.

3. Obstructed meridians. Blood circulates through the viscera to the back. An

accumulation of fever in the viscera lessens circulation of blood and as a result, fever toxin accumulates in the back and forms an abscess. Back pain ensues.

4. Pain caused by a fall or external injury. Impure, stagnated blood in the veins or arteries obstructs *ch'i* and manifests as bruising. Sometimes severe low back pain or a backache develops. Treatment calls for a circulatory agent along with an antidistress agent such as *tang-kuei* or peony.

5. Obstruction of lung *ch'i*. Chest distress, wheezing, or a chronic cough may cause a backache.

6. Weak blood vessels. Overexertion, prolonged sitting, or weak blood vessels also make the back ache.

Pain in the Hands and Feet

The pain arises when the flow of *ch'i* or blood is obstructed or insufficient or when sputum accumulates. Subsequently, the muscles and bones begin to atrophy. Conformations that involve pain in the hands and feet, including the elbows and arms, knees and legs, or ankles and shins, follow.

1. Chills caused by infection (influenza). Symptoms are aching in the hands and feet, pain and swelling in the legs and arms, a stiff neck, and severe chills.

2. Accumulation of wet toxin. Pain of rheumatic origin indicates its nature through gradual swelling of the feet and their growing weakness and numbness. The patient has trouble walking as the problem worsens.

3. Rheumatism. Wet toxin and chill invading the lower warmer cause pain and swelling in one or both knees.

4. Phlegm. An accumulation of sputum may underlie migratory pain in the hands and feet. Treatment is the same as for somatic pain or shoulder and back pain.

5. Amyotrophy. Muscle tissue not properly nourished by the blood results in atrophy, difficulty bending or stretching at the articular joints, an underdeveloped body, feverish palms or feet, a reddish tongue, and a small, rapid pulse.

6. Weak kidneys and weak bones. Kidney-strengthening agents relieve aching pain in the tibia and fibula.

Lower Back Pain

Pain in the area near the waist often relates to the kidneys. It may be caused by the kidneys being injured by an outside toxin or by impaired kidney *ch'i*.

1. Kidney problems caused by chills. Low back pain due to influenza often originates with feelings of icy coldness at the waist.

2. Accumulation of wet toxin in the kidneys. Wet toxin accumulated at the lower warmer provokes slight pain below the waist and bloating due to edema.

3. Injury to the kidneys from overexertion. Overexertion for a long period of time impairs kidney *ch'i* and causes low back pain.

4. Kidney weakness. Low back pain may follow sexual excess or overwork, or reflect disorders of the abdominal organs. Kidney weakness also causes chronic pain in the waist and knees of old people.

5. Bruises and stagnant blood. Extravasated blood resulting from a fall--bruises--may cause low back pain. Stagnant blood-expelling drugs ease the problem.

Pain in the Ribs

Costal pain affecting one or both sides usually accompanies diseases of the liver or gallbladder but may also appear with diseases of the other viscera. Possible causes of the pain follow.

1. Inside fever of the liver and gallbladder. Inside fever in this case results from dysfunction of the liver or gallbladder. Therapy utilizes bupleurum-containing drugs.

2. Stagnant *ch'i*. Depression, melancholia, or anger induce stagnation of *ch'i*.

3. Indigestion. Food accumulated in the stomach or an overabundance of liver *ch'i* may obstruct digestion and hence cause costal pain.

4. Phlegm. Costal pain provoked by congestion requires expectorants for treatment.

5. Stagnant blood in the meridians. Pain in the ribs caused by stagnant blood in the liver calls for circulatory agents and drugs that expel stagnant blood.

Rheumatism

Wind and moisture disease has no Western medical equivalent but is generally equated with rheumatism. One of the first references to the disease appears in *Summaries of Household Remedies* which says it is an illness with generalized pain. Because wind and moisture are fighting each other, the patient feels severe bone and joint pain and has trouble bending or stretching. *The Yellow Emperor's Classic of Internal Medicine* places wind and moisture disease as one of the numb diseases, characterized by greater pain during cold or damp weather. The four types of numb disease follow.

1. Wind or mobile numbness refers to a sudden attack of rheumatism charac-

terized by fever with pain and swelling of the joints. Therapy expels wind and improves blood circulation. Also included in mobile numbness are attacks of migratory arthritic pain.

2. Chill or pain numbness refers to chronic rheumatism characterized by a normal temperature, sporadic joint pain becoming severe during cold weather, and localized pallor and chills in the affected area. Therapy dispels wind and moisture.

3. Moist, fixed numbness occurs at a fixed site although several joints may be affected simultaneously. Pain is severe, especially at the joints. Other symptoms are numbness of the skin and muscles, severe swelling of the limb joints, joint deformities, and muscle atrophy. Moisture is said to adhere to the surface of the muscle. Therapy expels moisture and improves blood circulation.

4. Heat-induced numbness is characterized by fever, mild chills, and swelling with burning pain in the joint during hot weather. Severe cases exhibit symptoms of high fever, thirst, irritability, and emotional instability. Therapy dispels wind and heat.

Hypertension

Ancient Chinese medical texts contain detailed descriptions of hypertension and related symptoms such as headaches, vertigo, liver hyperfunction, apoplexy induced by liver toxin, and cerebral apoplexy. Today recognized symptoms are a big pulse, disharmony in *ch'i* and blood, increased liver hyperfunction, vertigo, palpitations, a tense pulse, and thin, white or dark red tongue fur. The disease is debilitating and the afflicted progress from firmness to weakness. The following symptoms identify each stage.

1. Liver fever: headaches, a feeling of pressure in the head, vertigo, ruddy complexion, dry mouth, red eyes, constipation, thirst, physical firmness, mental instability, irritability with severe fever, dry yellow tongue fur, a tense and strong pulse

2. Yin weakness and yang firmness: vertigo, dizziness, a feeling of heaviness in the head, tinnitus, irritability, numb arms and legs, trembling hands, red tongue, thin white tongue fur, a tense and small pulse

3. Yin weakness of the liver and kidneys: vertigo, dizziness, tinnitus, lumbago and weak legs, nocturia, weak *ch'i*, nocturnal emissions, impotence, no tongue fur, a sunken and small pulse, weakness of the deep pulse

4. Yin and yang weakness: the same symptoms as yin weakness of the liver and kidneys plus chillphobia, cold arms and legs, palpitations, shortness of breath, chest distress, diarrhea, a pale or red tongue without fur, a knotted and uneven pulse

5. Apoplexy: hemiplegia, unilateral facial paralysis, numb arms and legs, dizziness, difficulty turning the body

Hypotension

Hypotension may be substantial or symptomatic. Symptomatic hypotension often associates with psychosomatic complaints such as fatigue, weakness, neurosis, indigestion, and vertigo. The pulse is slow and weak. Substantial hypotension belongs to diseases of paralysis. It results from circulatory disorders caused by inadequate blood vessel function. The same herbal formula treats hypotension and hypertension because it adjusts imbalance. Along the same lines, the same herbs that treat stomach prolapse treat patients with hypotension and digestive problems.

Chills

Chills result mainly from weakness due to anemia, edema with hyperemia, and water intoxication. They may be accompanied by flushing and moderate fever in the limbs. Conditions with chills often herald gynecological problems but there are exceptions.

Palpitations

Chinese medicine concentrates not only on the unduly rapid pulse but also on throbbing and pulsating in other parts of the body. Palpitations may evidence themselves over the heart, abdomen, or umbilicus. They are a weak symptom but if associated with other complaints need not be considered essential to therapy.

Impotence

Traditionally, impotence is related to the liver, kidney, and sunlight yang meridians. It can result from sexual excess; worry and fright; injuries to the heart, spleen, or kidneys; or a downward moist fever. Impotence is classified according to the following accompanying symptoms.

1. Weakness of the right kidney: a pale complexion, vertigo and dizziness, lower back pain, aching and weakness of the legs, mental weakness, diluted semen, and a

sunken and small pulse without vigor

2. Deficiency of both heart and spleen: a chlorotic complexion, loss of appetite, fatigue, and weary arms and legs

3. Injury to the kidney from fright leading to emotional distress: fright and doubt, palpitations, and insomnia

4. Downward moist fever: feverish, ruddy urine; sticky, yellow fur on the tongue; and a soft, quick pulse

Hysteria

Called *tsang-tsao* (visceral agitation), hysteria is characterized by lack of control over behavior and emotions, morbid self-consciousness, anxiety, and psychosomatic manifestations. One specific complaint is *yen chung luen*—the sensation of a ball-shaped object rising from the stomach to the throat (hysteric ball). This symptom commonly accompanies menopausal disorders. Extremely nervous women may complain of stiffness or hardness of the lower left abdomen with the feeling of something rushing from the abdomen up to the throat. The woman may become so frightened that she feels faint and hyperventilates. This is called the "running pig" syndrome because a frightened running pig usually is panting. The underlying cause of all neurotic symptoms, however, is distress of *ch'i* or violent mental distress.

Eye Disease

Eye problems arise because of four possible reasons—water toxins, extravasated blood, food toxins, and congenital toxins. They belong to either an inner or outer conformation. The outer eye conformation includes inflammation of the eyelids, redness, swelling, pain, red-colored hyperemia (strong conformation), violet-colored hyperemia (extravasated blood), tearing (water toxins), and pale eyes with moderate inflammation (weak conformation). The inner eye conformation includes diseases of the inner eye and can be either strong or weak. The strong eye conformation covers disease caused by water toxin, extravasated blood, disturbed *ch'i*, and food toxin while the weak conformation covers eye disease caused by water toxin (the later stage), extravasated blood (the later stage), and weak blood. Most people with inner eye problems caused by disorders of the vitreous humor belong to the weak conformation.

Chronic Constipation

Chinese physicians pinpoint a number of possible causes for constipation—a dry fever accumulated inside, loss of fluid, overexcitement, stagnant *ch'i*, fatigue and internal injury, and insufficient blood and *ch'i*. The surrounding conformation may be strong or weak according to cause and symptoms.

Strong constipation subdivides into heat constipation and *ch'i* constipation. Symptoms of heat constipation are a ruddy face; fever; dry mouth and lips, bad breath, and a bitter taste in the mouth; a smooth, solid pulse; and yellow fur on the tongue with or without dryness. *Ch'i* constipation results from stagnation of liver *ch'i* and malcirculation of *ch'i*. Symptoms are frequent belching, hardness and distress over the heart and abdomen, chest distress and hardness, decrease in appetite, a tense pulse, and a thin tongue with heavy fur.

Weak constipation is classified as *ch'i* weakness, blood weakness, and chill constipation. *Ch'i* weakness results in difficulty moving the bowels despite normal stools; shortness of breath; a weak, soft pulse; and a light-colored tongue. Blood weakness constipation results in a pale face and lips. It is an anemic conformation. Other symptoms in addition to constipation are vertigo, palpitations, thin tongue fur, and a soft, small pulse. Chill constipation results in burning pain over the abdomen, difficult bowel movements, abundant and transparent urine, fondness of warmth, a light tongue with white fur, and a sunken, late pulse.

Chapter Nine

Properties and Actions of Herbal Drugs

Centuries of empirical knowledge of the medicinal properties of herbs have led Chinese theorists to suggest laws regarding the correspondence of drug action to the physical characteristics of the drugs themselves. Taste and color provide the most reliable indicators of specific action. Herbs most effective on diseases of the lungs and large intestine are white in color and have a pungent taste. Red, bitter herbs affect the heart and small intestine. Similarly, yellow, sweet drugs treat the stomach and spleen; black, salty drugs, the kidneys and bladder; and blue, sour drugs, the liver and gallbladder. These correspondences comprise part of the *wu hsing* or Five Element Theory.

Since Chinese doctors feel that disease is caused by changes in the equilibrium between yin and yang, drugs aim to adjust any imbalance. Complementary opposites, yin and yang, attract drugs to either pole of the body. Yin drugs, cold or cool, sink to the lower half of the body. Hot or warm yang drugs float upward to the thorax and head. The upper parts of plants, especially the flowers and leaves, are yang and light while the seeds, fruit, and roots are yin and heavy. For example, if a patient suffers from a yang fever, he is treated with a yin cool drug. A yin cool problem requires a yang warm drug.

The properties of drugs include four essences, five flavors, and four directions of action. The four essences are cool, warm, cold, and hot. A cool drug alleviates yang diseases, inflammation or hyperemia, and various fevers. Hot drugs heat yin problems such as "cool water intoxication." If yang fever diseases are treated with hot drugs or yin chill diseases with cold drugs, the condition worsens. For example, gypsum is cold; aconite, hot; cassia, warm; and pueraria, cool.

Hot, sour, sweet, bitter, and salty are the five flavors. A drug's flavor indicates its pharmacological action. A hot-tasting drug, such as ginger, mint, or schizonepeta, disperses or eliminates toxins from the body. Orange peel, cyperus, and amomum are hot herbs and promote flowing, thus encouraging good circulation. Sour drugs astringe and absorb. For instance, *Chebulae fructus, Granati pericarpium*, and Chinese gall treat diarrhea and prolapse of the rectum, and schizandra fruit and *Rosae fructus* reduce sweating and enhance energy. Sweet drugs, such as rehmannia and ophiopogon, are tonics and supplement warm drugs. Ginseng and astragalus supplement or reinforce body strength while licorice and maltose moderate the unpleasant tastes of the other herbs. Bitter drugs dry and purge the body. Examples are coptis and phellodendron, which reduce sensations of heat, and rhubarb, which warms as it purges. Salty drugs soften and lubricate. Thus sargassum thins thick sputum and sodium sulfate quenches thirst and moistens. Tasteless or bland drugs, such as hoelen and tetrapanax, are diuretics.

According to *The Yellow Emperor's Classic of Internal Medicine*, the five flavors relate to the five visceral organs: hot to the lungs; sour to the liver; sweet to the spleen; bitter to the heart; and salty to the kidneys. Thus hot herbs relieve lung distress and sweet herbs supplement weakness of the spleen and stomach. Herbs for the liver are soaked in an acetic acid solution and those for the kidneys in salty water.

Other factors further determine the actions of drugs. The flavors are either yin or yang in nature–sour, bitter, and salty belonging to yin and pungent, sweet, and tasteless to yang. Furthermore, drugs of the same flavor often differ in essence or vice versa. For instance, ginger is pungent and warm while magnolia is bitter and warm; astragalus, sweet and warm; mume, sour and warm; and gecko, salty and warm. Gypsum is acrid and cold; aconite, acrid and hot; mentha, acrid and cool. Therefore, to fully understand the function of a drug, one must know its flavor, essence, and nature. Complicated aspects of the disease itself must also be considered. For example, an outside fever requires a hot-tasting, but cool, sweating agent whereas an inside strong fever requires a bitter or salty, cold purgative. Any drug given without considering the four essences and five flavors will cause the disease to worsen.

In addition to the essence, flavor, and nature of herbs, the direction of the actions of drugs influences prescriptions. Ascending and floating drugs rise, move outwards, expel, and are yang in nature; descending and sinking drugs move inward and are astringent, diuretic, and yin in nature.

Generally, sweet drugs, such as cinnamon and ginger, float and ascend, and hot and sour drugs, such as rhubarb, peony, sodium sulfate, and oyster shell sink and descend. Similarly, light drugs, such as mentha leaf, cinnamon, magnolia, and cimicifuga, also float and ascend, and herbs with heavy seeds and fruits, such as citrus, rehmannia, and magnetite, descend and sink. Ascending yang diseases exhibit headaches and dizziness and are treated with descending *Hallotidis concha* and oyster shell while chronic descending problems, such as diarrhea or prolapse of the rectum, are treated with ascending ginseng, astragalus, and cimicifuga.

In sum then, clinical application follows a heteropathic course. Hot or warm drugs attack cold conditions, and cold or cool drugs, hot conditions; light, floating drugs treat conditions of the lower body and heavy sinking drugs counteract problems in the upper body and head. Thus these general guidelines following the natural laws of the universe dictate the formulation of remedies.

The Seven Effects of Drugs

Early physicians found that the effects of single herbs change with their herbal environment. Some combinations enhance an action while other combinations become toxic. Seven possible effects of drugs follow.

1. Singular. A drug with one component produces one effect.

2. Additive. Two or more drugs with the same physiological effects retain their respective effects when combined, such as anemarrhena and phellodendron.

3. Synergic. Two or more drugs with different physiological effects become more efficient when combined, such as hoelen and astragalus.

4. Antagonistic. Two or more drugs with different physiological effects when combined depress one another's effects, such as pinellia and ginger.

5. Inhibitive. One drug may inhibit the effect of another, such as ginger and scute.

6. Destructive. Two drugs combined become less toxic than when used separately, such as siler and arsenic.

7. Opposite. Two drugs combined become more toxic and cause violent side effects, such as aconite and pinellia.

Incompatibilities of Drugs

Care must be exercised in preparation and consumption of drugs to prevent incompatibilities. For example, cyperus and tree peony decocted in an iron container produce side effects, as do rehmannia and scrophularia decocted in a copper container. Furthermore, people taking drugs should not eat foods of opposing taste, odor, or properties. For example, people taking warm drugs should avoid cool or cold foods; those taking digestives should avoid fatty foods that inhibit digestion; those taking sedatives should avoid stimulating foods. Similarly, to avoid harming her unborn child, a pregnant woman should never take violent-acting drugs such as peach seeds, carthamus, *chih-shih*, rhubarb, and aconite, or toxic drugs such as croton and *Pharbitidis semen*.

Classification of Drugs

1. **Sweating agents.** Mainly pungent and dispersing, they alleviate surface problems such as headaches, fever, and chills. One type disperses mild fevers and chills, headaches, thirst, and conjunctivitis; the other, severe chills with little fever and heart pain, in addition to the other symptoms.

2. **Emetics.** Because they are toxic, they should not be taken by pregnant and postpartum women. They treat a sore throat, sputum disturbances in the chest, overeating, and intoxication.

3. **Purgatives.** These eliminate accumulated food and dry stools. Violent purgatives treat serious constipation. Moderate purgatives lubricate.

4. **Diuretics.** These treat excretory problems such as peripheral edema, abdominal swelling, vomiting, and difficult urination. Diuretics per se are moderate drugs, but certain expelling agents are violent and not recommended for people of weak and yin conformations. Expelling agents treat general edema and sputum disturbances.

5. **Antirheumatics.** Inadvisable for yin weak or anemic people, these are always taken in conjunction with sweating agents. Rheumatism—commonly caused by living in low, wet areas—exhibits primary symptoms of chills, fever, exhaustion, dizziness, stiffness, and swollen joints. In severe conditions, the pain spreads from the joints and becomes generalized.

6. **Cold agents.** Not recommended for yin, weak people or those with fevers, these are pungent, warm, and dry. They treat common cold symptoms, vomiting, diarrhea, abdominal pain, a slow pulse, and pale complexion.

7. **Refreshing agents.** These clean and detoxify the blood in people whose surface fever has been dispersed but who still suffer from systemic fever. In excess, they are toxic and harm the stomach and pancreas. Obviously they must be used with caution by those with impaired function of these organs. One type of refreshing agent disperses heat and is suitable for people with fever, thirst, diarrhea, jaundice, and ulcers; the other refreshes the blood in people suffering from convulsions, diarrhea, measles, and smallpox.

8. **Antitussives and expectorants.** These stop coughing and stimulate sputum

production respectively. Antitussives treat asthma by facilitating expectoration of thick (hot) mucus and excessive sputum.

9. Distress agents. These suppress symptoms caused by inclement weather, overeating, and anxiety. Mostly pungent, warm, and dry, and of various flavors, anti-distress agents act as analgesics and improve digestion. They are not recommended for yin weak people.

10. Blood agents. Tonics and styptics treat anemia and hyperemia; styptics alone treat bloody stools, hematuria, and hemoptysis; and extravasated blood agents treat extravasated blood, menstrual irregularities, abdominal swelling and pain, stomach or intestinal ulcers, contusions, and pancreatic disorders.

11. Tonics. These benefit weak patients but only if no toxins are in the body.

12. Inhalants. For syncope, unconsciousness, and high fevers, except where heavy sweating and vomiting are present, these stimulate breathing.

13. Tranquilizers. These reduce anxiety and its accompanying symptoms: palpitations and insomnia. They also ease convulsions and cramps according to the type of drug. People with mental instability who have lost blood should take tonics in addition to tranquilizers. Refreshing agents help promote mental stability in people with fever.

14. Astringents. These treat prolapse of the rectum and excessive excreta. One type treats sweating; the other, diarrhea.

15. Digestive agents. For abdominal pain and loss of appetite.

16. Anthelmintics. These kill parasites, thereby reducing abdominal swelling and pain.

17. External medicines, ointments, balms, and sprays. Generally toxic if taken internally, they have local rather than systemic effects.

The actual chemical components of most herbs have yet to be determined. Some, such as ma-huang, have been found to contain certain elements present in Western commercial drugs. More studies in the future will add to the knowledge of the properties and actions of the herbs.

Chapter Ten

An Overview of Prescriptions

Names of Formulas

Formulas are named in several ways. Sometimes an herb in the formula gives its name to the compound. This is particularly true of major herbs. Other formulas take their names from the symptoms that they treat. Oddly, some formulas containing the same components go under different names. Others are known only by their abbreviations. Any reduction or addition to a formula may appear in the name as may the number or kind of components included, the combination of two formulas, origin of the prescription, dosage, and form (liquid, powder, or tablet).

Structure of Formulas

The structure of a formula revolves around four types of herbs: imperial (*chun*), ministerial (*chen*), assistant (*tso*), and servant (*shih*). The major ingredient is called the emperor. The subsidiary ingredient–the minister–assists the emperor by promoting its action. The assistant lessens the imperial herb's side effects or limits its actions, particularly if the imperial herb possesses toxic properties. The servant renders the formula more palatable. Ma-huang Combination is a good example. In this formula, ma-huang, a sudorific, takes the part of the imperial herb. Cinnamon–the minister–

also promotes sweating. Apricot seed, the assistant, lessens ma-huang's antitussive effects and licorice gives the concoction a pleasant taste. Different herb combinations produce different effects, however. For example, ma-huang with apricot seed eases coughing, but ma-huang with atractylodes promotes urination for treatment of dysuria, edema, and lack of sweating. Both ma-huang and cinnamon, and ma-huang and gypsum, promote sweating.

Classification of Formulas

The Yellow Emperor's Classic of Internal Medicine outlined a system for combining drugs based upon the number and type of herbs. Contemporary physicians certainly do not restrict themselves to this system. Indeed, following generations published extensive discussions on methods of altering formula components. For instance, Chang Chung-ching in *Treatise on Febrile Diseases* described 86 herbs and 130 combinations and modified dosages to treat different illnesses according to the symptoms.

Over time Chinese herbal prescriptions have been classified according to a number of different systems. One system still in use originated in ancient times. It incorporates parts of *The Yellow Emperor's Classic* system. Its basic rules are these:

Large prescription: for grave illnesses of two or more concurrent conformations that require immediate care

Small prescription: for light and shallow illnesses without a concurrent conformation. Used in small doses

Moderating prescription: for long term use in such illnesses as a weak fever conformation

Urgent prescription: for acute conformations that worsen without prompt treatment

Odd prescription: for illnesses of simple cause that can be cured by a single drug. The prescription contains only one drug

Even prescription: for more complicated illnesses. Combines two drugs

Complex prescription: a mixture of three or more drugs

Another system originated during the Tang dynasty with Chen Tsang-chi. He classified prescriptions into ten groups: *husan* formulas remove fullness, *tung* clear stagnancy, *pu* supplement weakness, *hsieh* open closed spaces, *ching* diminish strong forces, *chung* ease anxiety, *hua* eliminate stickiness, *se* free immoveable concentrations, *tsao* dry wetness, *shih* moisten dryness.

During the Ming dynasty, Chang Ching-yueh arranged prescriptions into eight classes corresponding to the eight methods of treatment. *Pu* formulas supplement loss of vigor and delicate health. *Ho* harmonize the body. *Kung* attack acute illness in people of strong conformation. *San* suit an outside conformation. *Han* warm a cold conformation but also lower heat. *Je* cool a fever conformation, strengthen yang, and lessen chilling. *Ku* promote free flow of fluids. *Yin* aid diagnosis according to the causes of illness.

Modern classification arose from the Ching dynasty's *I fang chi chieh* edited by Wang Ang. It puts prescriptions into twenty-three categories.

1. **Tonics** supplement weakness and debility by nourishing blood, *ch'i*, yin, and yang. Four Major Herb Combination supplements *ch'i;* Tang-kuei Four Combination or Tang-kuei and Astragalus Combination nourishes yin; Ginseng and Longan Combination supplements blood and the lungs; and Rehmannia Six Formula fortifies yang.

2. **Sudorifics** promote sweating, disperse external toxins, and treat surface conformations. They belong to one of three types: acrid warm; acrid cool; and lung. Ma-huang Combination and Cinnamon Combination are acrid warm sudorifics. Morus and Chrysanthemum Combination and Lonicera and Forsythia Formula are acrid cool sudorifics. Cyperus and Perilla Formula is a lung sudorific. Acrid cool sudorifics prove more effective against pulmonary disorders or coughs while Lonicera and Forsythia Formula reduces surface fevers. A lung sudorific more effectively treats obstructed *ch'i* and the *ch'i* conformation caused by a surface toxin.

3. **Emetics** induce vomiting as a means of removing injurious toxins. The representative formula is Melon Pedicel Formula.

4. **Interior attacking formulas,** such as Major Rhubarb Combination, are laxatives that clean out obstructions and accumulations in the stomach and intestines. Minor Rhubarb Combination also belongs to this type. The difference between the two formulas lies in the former's greater amount of rhubarb, resulting in a more violent action. It thus treats obstruction, distention, dryness, and firmness. The latter, with its lighter dose of rhubarb, treats only obstruction, distention, and firmness.

5. **Surface and interior attacking formulas,** as implied by the name, treat both the outside and the inside of the human body. For example, in Cinnamon and Rhubarb Combination, cinnamon combats external toxins while rhubarb battles internal ones. Another example is Siler and Platycodon Formula, which lowers a fever.

6. **Harmonizing formulas,** like Minor Bupleurum Combination, generally harmonize the body by removing toxins. They are appropriate when the patient has entered the lesser yang stage and cannot be treated by sweating, vomiting, or purging agents. Other examples are Tang-kuei and Bupleurum Formula and Coptis Combination.

7. ***Ch'i* formulas** dissolve *ch'i* stagnation, cause *ch'i* and adverse upflushing

73

of *ch'i* to descend, and replenish *ch'i*. Symptoms are obstruction and depression below the chest, swelling pain, distention, vomiting, nausea, heartburn, *ch'i* adversity, and asthma. Representative formulas are Inula and Hematite Combination, Pinellia and Magnolia Combination, and Perilla Fruit Combination.

8. **Blood formulas** remove occluded blood, stop bleeding, and promote the replenishment of the blood. Occluded blood means extravasation or stagnation occurring in ordinary injuries. Acute, spontaneous symptoms with distention, extravasation, pain, fainting, and mania generally call for formulas that attack the extravasated or occluded blood, such as Persica and Rhubarb Combination. Trachycarpus and Biota Leaf Formula and Sophora Flower Formula stop bleeding.

9. **Carminatives,** or wind-dispelling formulas, are differentiated between external and internal wind conformations. "External wind" results from penetration of the body by an external toxin. When serious it is known as wind stroke and characterized by unconsciousness, convulsions of the muscles or vessels, contractions of the eyes and mouth, and blurred speech. "Internal wind" resembles "external wind" but further exhibits partial paralysis, slobbering, and spasms of the mouth. However, the chief distinction between the two lies in the failure of the internal wind conformation to exhibit any symptoms along the six meridians. Wind diseases must be treated with a carminative. Wind-dispelling formulas are represented by Ma-huang and Paeonia Combination and Tu-huo and Vaeicum Combination. Rehmannia Combination nourishes the kidneys and removes wet phlegm, thus treating wind conformation too.

10. **Chill-dispelling formulas** chiefly warm and nourish. Representative formulas are Aconite, Ginger, and Licorice Combination; Vitality Combination; and Evodia Combination.

11. **Heat-dispelling formulas**–such as Talc and Licorice Formula, Cardamon Formula, Agastache Formula, and Astragalus and Atractylodes Combination–treat summer conditions such as heatstroke.

12. **Moisture-dispelling formulas** encourage excretion. Moisture can be either internal or external. External moisture refers to ailments due to sweat, rain, or humidity in which liquid toxins invade the body through the open pores. In internal moisture disease, fluids accumulate from excessive intake of water, fruit, and alcohol causing abnormal spleen and stomach functioning. The liquid toxins materialize internally. Moist toxins in the upper body cause headaches and dizziness; on the surface, chills and fever, generalized heaviness and aching, and edema in the arms and legs; in the interior of the middle of the torso, chest paralysis, vomiting, stomach distention, abdominal fullness, or jaundice; and in the lower body, swelling in the leg muscles and turbid urine.

Sudorifics dispel fluid in the upper body and on the surface. Stomachics, diuretics, and spleen-strengthening formulas eliminate fluid in the lower and middle body. In prescribing formulas, however, attention must be paid to whether the condition is cold or hot in nature. For example, a wet chill calls for acrid, warm, and dry herbs–such as atractylodes, magnolia, and citrus peel–while hot conditions call for bitter, cool, and dry herbs–such as coptis, scute, and phellodendron. Severe fluid stagnation that causes edema must be treated according to weakness or firmness of the conformation. Edema in a person with a firm pulse and strong build requires water-dispelling methods. On the other hand, a weak person with a submerged and slow pulse requires formulas that strengthen the spleen, such as Hoelen Five Herb Formula, Polyporus Combination, Areca and Hoelen Combination, Jujube Combination, Atractylodes and Hoelen Combination, and Capillaris Combination. Both Hoelen Five Herb Formula and Polyporus Combination are diuretics. They treat water stagnation in a yin weak person or one with dysuria. Hoelen Five Herb Formula eases dysuria, a dry mouth, and regurgitation. Areca and Hoelen Combination treats edema. Jujube Combination is a strong diuretic. Capillaris Combination reduces fevers, helps dispel moisture, and treats jaundice.

13. **Moistening formulas** wash away externally contracted dry toxins, nourish swollen abdomens, stimulate saliva production, and increase body fluids. Diseases of aridity can be either external or internal in nature. External dryness further divides into warm and cool. In late autumn the weather becomes cool and the western winds stop blowing. A cold caught at this time exhibits symptoms of cool aridity, whereas a cold caught on a clear, dry, warm autumn day is characterized by warm aridity symptoms. Cool aridity usually affects the lungs, resulting in a cough, stuffy nose, headaches, chillphobia, and dry lips. Warm aridity also attacks the lungs but causes headache, discomfort, generalized fever, a dry cough, scanty saliva, a dry mouth, and stagnation. Thin, white fur appears on the tongue of which the apex and rim are red and the other areas white. A lack of internal fluid (dehydration) is serious. Aridity in the upper body causes the nose and throat to dry out; in the middle of the body, thirst; and in the lower body, constipation. The rule of treatment is to restore saliva for upper aridity, promote fluid production for middle aridity, and nourish the blood for lower aridity. Representative formulas are Cyperus and Perilla Formula for cool aridity and Eriobotrya and Ophiopogon Combination for warm aridity.

14. **Fire-purging formulas** reduce heat, cool the blood, or detoxify. They divide into four groups: fire-cleansing formulas acting on *ch'i*; fire-cleansing formulas acting on blood; fire-cleansing formulas for restoring *ch'i* and blood; and miscellaneous fire-cleansing formulas.

Fire purgatives which act on *ch'i* are Gypsum Combination, Bamboo Leaf and Gypsum Combination, Coptis and Scute Combination, and Forsythia and Rhubarb

Formula. Gypsum Combination is an acrid, cold febrifuge for strong fever and extreme thirst. Bamboo Leaf and Gypsum Combination is a sweet, acrid, cool fire purgative with stronger stomachic and saliva-producing actions than Gypsum Combination. Coptis and Scute Combination is a bitter, cold fire purgative. Forsythia and Rhubarb Formula cleanses a fever and promotes bowel movements.

Fire purgatives which act on blood, such as Rhinoceros and Rehmannia Combination, attack fever toxins that have invaded the blood. The conformation is marked by high fever, depression, hallucinations, and other symptoms.

Fire-cleansing formulas for excessive *ch'i* and blood are represented by Rehmannia and Gypsum Combination, Gypsum and Moutan Combination, and Scute and Cimicifuga Combination—all modifications of Gypsum Combination. They are for conditions in which a fever attacks the *ch'i* and blood. They cleanse the blood and remove stomach fever and are prescribed for contagious diseases, toothaches, hemoptysis, and nosebleeds.

15. Expectorants render removal of sputum or phlegm. Sputum diseases involve congestion and often rise and fall with *ch'i*. For instance, ascending *ch'i* brings on asthma and coughing whereas descending *ch'i* causes diarrhea. Ascending *ch'i* also induces dizziness, vomiting, cardiac palpitations, or epilepsy.

Sputum may be wet or dry. Injuries to the spleen cause fluid to transform into wet sputum while insufficiency of liver yin changes fluid into dry sputum. Feverish congestion is called hot sputum whereas chilled congestion is called cold sputum. Sputum resulting from food stagnation is called food sputum and sputum due to the imbalance of *ch'i* is called obstructed sputum. Thus treatment for sputum disorders depends on the cause. For food sputum, digestives are indicated and for obstructed sputum, *ch'i*-dissolving expectorants. Two chief formulas are Citrus and Pinellia Combination and Ginseng, Atractylodes, and Licorice Formula.

16. Aromatic inhalants restore consciousness in people who have passed out principally because of fever toxin trapped within the heart or sputum and saliva lodged in the throat. Such formulas induce expectoration. Representative formulas are Bos and Musk Formula and Bos and Curcuma Formula.

17. Sedatives and spasmolytics include all combinations that possess tranquilizing and convulsion-arresting actions. They are generally used for cardiac palpitations, insomnia, amnesia, hallucinations, epilepsy, and convulsions. Representative formulas are Ginseng and Zizyphus Formula and Zizyphus Combination.

18. Digestives dissolve accumulations, aid digestion, and strengthen spleen and stomach functions. Representative formulas are Magnolia and Ginger Formula; Ginseng, Coptis, and Atractylodes Formula; and Crataegus and Citrus Formula.

19. Astringents astringe semen and *ch'i* and stop excessive production of saliva and body fluids. Prolonged illnesses in people with weak physiques or excessive use of attacking herbs may cause oversecretion of fluids resulting in spontaneous sweating, night sweats, and spermatorrhea in men; incontinence, frequent urination, and metrorrhagia in women—symptoms all treated with astringents. There are three types of astringents: intestinal, anhidrotic, and spermatostatic. The chief ones are Kaolin and Oryza Combination, Oyster Shell Formula, and Lotus Stamen Formula.

20. Anthelmintics dispel parasites from the stomach and intestines of an infested patient. Symptoms are a pale facial complexion with white spots, red or white spots in the mouth or on the lips, cardiac irregularity and abdominal pain, vomiting of water, grinding of the teeth, mental fatigue, and loss of appetite. Representative formulas are Mume Formula, Picrorrhiza and Mume Combination, and Quisqualis Formula.

21. Vision-improving formulas treat ophthalmic diseases. Eye diseases generally derive from visceral disorders. For example, excessive heart fire causes mydriasis (abnormal dilation of the pupil) and should be treated with a blood-nourishing and fire-purging formula. Eye diseases due to weakness in the liver, kidneys, or *ch'i* should be treated by a liver-replenishing and kidney-nourishing formula. Representative formulas are Rehmannia and Cornus Formula, Hoelen and Polygala Formula, and Cnidium and Chrysanthemum Formula.

22. Carbuncle and dermatosis formulas are applied externally or internally. Skin ailments that are red, swollen, aching, and burning are called *yung* (carbunculosis) and require treatment of the skin and body surface and inducement of bowel movements if constipation exists. White, painless, progressive induration is called *chu* (ulcer) and in most cases belongs to the yin conformation. Chief formulas are Angelica and Mastic Combination, Cimicifuga and Gleditsia Combination, and Rhubarb and Moutan Combination.

23. Obstetric and gynecological formulas treat abnormal menstruation, leukorrhea, and problems of pregnancy and childbirth. Chief formulas are Gelatin and Artemisia Combination, Tang-kuei and Evodia Combination, and Tang-kuei and Paeonia Formula.

As has been said, herbal doctors prescribe formulas according to conformation. Sometimes they alter basic formulas to fit individual needs, for example, adding or deleting rhubarb according to the presence or absence of constipation. The next Chapter delineates formula conformations and Chapter Twelve gives the ingredients and indications of 68 basic formulas.

Chapter Eleven

A List of Formulas
According to Conformation

This chapter lists the many formulas of Chinese medicine and their corresponding conformations. However, since the Western reader is more familiar with diseases and symptoms, the formulas have been arranged accordingly. The first part covers diseases and the second part common symptoms. Because of this arrangement, formulas are repeated under the different headings.

Part 1: Preferred Medication for Various Diseases

I. Diseases of the Respiratory System

Common Cold

Pueraria Combination

A cold without sweating but with a chilled and feverish feeling; stiff shoulders, neck, back, and legs; headache

Ma-huang Combination

Aching joints, body pain, headache, cough, stuffy nose, and any of the symp-

toms of Pueraria Combination. In general it treats influenza and nasal congestion in children.

Minor Blue Dragon Combination

Coughing with thin sputum and asthmatic breathing, occasional chest pain,
excessive urination

Bupleurum and Cinnamon Combination

Sweating with persistent moderate fever; cold, severe chills; upper respiratory
infection

Minor Bupleurum Combination

Prolonged cold with cough and moderate fever, bitter taste in mouth and loss
of appetite

Pinellia and Magnolia Combination

Throat and chest distress and dry cough

Cyperus and Perilla Formula

Headache, melancholia, and loss of appetite in delicate females and elderly
patients who are unable to take Ma-huang Combination

Bronchitis, Whooping Cough, Bronchial
and Childhood Asthma, and Bronchial Dilation

Minor Blue Dragon Combination

Asthmatic breathing with copious, thin sputum; chest pain; bronchial dilation

Ma-huang and Apricot Combination

Severe cough, head sweating, and thirst; childhood asthma

Ma-huang Combination

Same symptoms as Ma-huang and Apricot Combination but without sweating.
May be given to infants.

Ophiopogon Combination

Severe cold or very sticky sputum that is difficult to expectorate

Pinellia and Magnolia Combination

Thirst, distress from the throat to the chest, sensation of distention, labored breathing, psychoneurotic behavior

Ma-huang and Magnolia Combination

Same complaints as Ma-huang and Apricot Combination and Ma-huang Combination except with bronchial asthma. Prolonged use required.

Minor Bupleurum Combination with Pinellia and Magnolia Combination

Poorly controlled bronchial asthma unresponsive to para-adrenalin or ephedrine; chronic chest or abdominal distress. Prolonged use of both formulas required.

Major Bupleurum Combination with Pinellia and Magnolia Combination

Same symptoms as Minor Bupleurum Combination and Pinellia and Magnolia Combination with heart distress and constipation

Bupleurum and Scute Combination

Chest pain, excessive sputum, gastric distress, bronchial dilation

Tuberculosis and Pleurisy

Minor Bupleurum Combination

Loss of appetite, moderate fever, weakness, stiff shoulders and back

Ginseng and Astragalus Combination

More severe symptoms than Minor Bupleurum Combination; given with chemotherapy during recovery periods to provide additional nutrients

Bupleurum and Cinnamon Combination

Moderate fever, chest or abdominal pain, night sweats

Bupleurum, Cinnamon, and Ginger Combination

Marked weakness, insomnia, palpitation, night sweats, thirst, a tendency toward soft stools

Ophiopogon Combination

Severe cough with thick sputum (sometimes bloody) and an occasional flushing sensation

Bupleurum and Scute Combination

The same symptoms as Ophiopogon Combination along with pulmonary edema or chest pain

Minor Blue Dragon Combination

Pulmonary edema, chest pain, thin sputum, occasional moderate fever

Ginseng Nutritive Combination

Chronic cough or moderate fever with delicate health

Coptis and Scute Formula

Mental instability, flushing with expectoration of blood in patients unresponsive to chemotherapy. It is more effective if given with Minor Bupleurum Combination.

Tang-kuei and Gelatin Combination

More severe coughing of blood than Coptis and Scute Formula conformation with anemia and menstrual irregularity

Cinnamon and Hoelen Formula

Expectoration of blood, vicarious or difficult menstruation

Magnolia and Ginger Formula

Gastrointestinal disturbances or loss of appetite due to continuous use of para-aminosalicylic acid

Pinellia Combination

Abdominal pain and soft stools or diarrhea along with symptoms of Magnolia and Ginger Formula

II. Diseases of the Digestive System

Stomatitis, Gastritis, Impaired Digestion, Prolapsed Stomach, Gastric Psychoneurosis, and Gastric Dilation

Coptis and Scute Formula

Stomatitis, inflammation of the lips and mouth

Cardamon and Fennel Formula

Chill conformation, psychoneurosis, stomach pain or heart distress

Magnolia and Ginger Formula

Indigestion, stomachache, vomiting after eating

Pinellia Combination

Nausea, vomiting, gastric distress with a tendency toward diarrhea, soft stools, occasional constipation

Pinellia and Magnolia Combination

Poor digestion, prolapsed stomach, gastric neurosis, throat and chest distress due to psychoneurosis

Minor Bupleurum Combination

Loss of appetite, a tendency to tire, stiff shoulders, a white-coated tongue

Ginseng and Astragalus Combination

Malaise, impaired digestion, a tendency to tire, loss of appetite

Bupleurum and Cinnamon Combination

Severe stomach pain and cramps, nausea, cardiac distress

Major Bupleurum Combination

Heart distress and severe constipation

Hoelen Combination

Stomach distention with indigestion, cardiac hyperfunction, and gastric dilation

Major Zanthoxylum Combination

Cold abdomen and prolapse of the viscera with stomach pain

Minor Cinnamon and Paeonia Combination

Less severe symptoms than Major Zanthoxylum Combination. Especially good for stomachaches in children.

Gastric and Duodenal Ulcers

Cardamon and Fennel Formula

Chills, severe heart distress, nausea, stomach pain

Bupleurum and Cinnamon Combination

Severe stomach pain, nausea, vomiting, tension around the heart

Minor Bupleurum Combination

Chest or abdominal distress, loss of appetite, white tongue fur

Pinellia Combination

Stomach distress, nausea, vomiting, soft stools and diarrhea alternating with constipation

Minor Cinnamon and Paeonia Combination

Stomach pain resulting from loss of gastric acid

Major Bupleurum Combination

Angina and severe constipation

Siler and Platycodon Formula

Obesity, constipation, cardiac distress

Coptis and Scute Formula

Coughing of blood, bloody or soft stools, occasional constipation, flushing, mental instability

Coptis and Rhubarb Combination

Symptoms similar to Coptis and Scute Formula and bloody or hard stools with constipation

Hepatitis, Cirrhosis of the Liver, Jaundice, Cholecystitis, Cholelithiasis, and Pancreatitis

Major Bupleurum Combination

Liver disease, heart distress, constipation, pancreatitis

Minor Bupleurum Combination

Liver disease, chest or abdominal distress, proneness to fatigue, loss of appetite, pancreatitis

Minor Bupleurum Combination with Hoelen Five Herb Formula

Cirrhosis of the liver with ascites. When the patient also has cardiac distress and constipation, Minor Bupleurum Combination is more effective than Major Bupleurum Combination. Hepatitis, stones in the gallbladder or in a bile duct, inflammation of the gallbladder or pancreas, nausea, vomiting, and loss of appetite are also treated with these two formulas.

Minor Bupleurum Combination with Coptis and Scute Formula

Gastric distress caused by jaundice, moderate fever, loss of appetite

Capillaris Combination with Hoelen Five Herb Formula

Jaundice, thirst, thoracic distress with constipation

Bupleurum and Cinnamon Combination

Stones in the gallbladder or bile duct; inflammation of the gallbladder with slight pain and nausea

Hoelen Combination

Stones in the gallbladder or bile duct, inflammation of the gallbladder with slight pain, vomiting or cardiac hyperfunction

Bupleurum, Cinnamon, and Ginger Combination

Delicate health, head sweating, night sweats with hepatitis, inflammation of the pancreas or gallbladder, palpitation

Peritonitis and Appendicitis

Minor Bupleurum Combination

Peritonitis and chest or abdominal distress with loss of appetite. Hoelen Five Herb Formula is prescribed jointly if the patient has ascites.

Ginseng and Astragalus Combination

Peritonitis with proneness to fatigue greater than Minor Bupleurum Combination

Bupleurum, Cinnamon, and Ginger Combination
Peritonitis, palpitation, mental instability, insomnia because of poor health

Major Zanthoxylum Combination
Peritonitis, intestinal distention with abdominal pain

Minor Cinnamon and Paeonia Combination
Peritonitis and weakness but without ascites

Rhubarb and Moutan Combination
Acute appendicitis with ulceration and constipation. Discontinue if pain persists or patient feels discomfort. Eriocheir and Viper Formula may be prescribed jointly.

Major Zanthoxylum Combination
Subacute or chronic appendicitis, abdominal pain and distention, or hyperperistalsis

Bupleurum and Cinnamon Combination
Primary appendicitis and general abdominal pain

Cinnamon and Hoelen Formula with coix
Chronic appendicitis with minor pain when palpated, slow recovery

III. Diseases of the Circulatory System

Heart Diseases

Stephania and Ginseng Combination
Endocarditis, valvular disease, cardiac asthma; difficult breathing, cough, stridor, edema, thirst, chest distress

Bupleurum, Cinnamon, and Ginger Combination
Valvular disease, cardiac asthma; thoracic distress, palpitation, insomnia, soft stools, weakness

Ginseng and Tang-kuei Formula
Valvular disease, chills, anemia

Hoelen Five Herb Formula

Valvular disease, thirst, frequent urination with decreased volume, edema

Pinellia and Magnolia Combination

Diseases implicating the cardiac nerves and symptoms associated with cardiac hyperfunction

Atractylodes and Hoelen Combination

Palpitation, dizziness, unsteadiness with no evidence of cardiac failure

Bupleurum and Dragon Bone Combination

Angina pectoris, disorders of the cardiac nerves, cardiac asthma; palpitation, constipation, general weakness

Major Bupleurum Combination

Fatty or distressed heart with severe constipation

Siler and Platycodon Formula

Fatty heart and obesity with constipation

Hypertension, Arteriosclerosis, and Partial Paralysis

Coptis and Rhubarb Combination

Hypertension, arteriosclerosis, mental instability, flushing, stomach distress, constipation

Major Bupleurum Combination

Hypertension, arteriosclerosis, stiff shoulders, tinnitus, cardiac distress, constipation

Bupleurum and Dragon Bone Combination

Hypertension, arteriosclerosis, psychoneurosis with palpitation, chest distress, insomnia, constipation

Siler and Platycodon Formula

Obesity, hypertension, arteriosclerosis with constipation

Persica and Rhubarb Combination

Hypertension, arteriosclerosis, cold feet or waist, headache, constipation, lower abdominal pain

Rehmannia Eight Formula

Hypertension, arteriosclerosis, lower back pain, nocturia, thirst in elderly persons

Atractylodes and Hoelen Combination

Hypertension, headache, vertigo, palpitation, decreased urinary volume

Ginseng and Tang-kuei Formula

Hypertension, chills, a tendency towards anemia, dizziness, stiff shoulders, albuminuria with decreased urine volume and increased frequency

Cinnamon, Atractylodes, and Aconite Combination

Chills and partial paralysis following cerebral hemorrhage

Coptis and Scute Formula

Mental instability, flushing, and stomach distress in those who cannot take Coptis and Rhubarb Combination

Gastrodia and Gambir Combination

Hypertension, apoplexy

Complex Polygonum Combination

Hypertension, yin weakness of the liver and kidneys

Hypotension

Ginseng and Astragalus Combination

Malaise, a tendency toward anemia, loss of appetite, fatigue

Ginseng and Tang-kuei Formula

Chills, anemia, dizziness, stiff shoulders, frequent urination with decreased volume

Minor Cinnamon and Paeonia Combination

Hypotension, loss of vitality, fatigue

Atractylodes and Hoelen Combination

Headache, flushing, vertigo, cardiac hyperfunction with decreased urinary volume

Pinellia and Magnolia Combination

Heavy head and weakness

Tang-kuei and Paeonia Formula

Facial pallor and cold limbs in women

Pueraria Combination

Cold and numb limbs, impaired motion, pain

IV. Genito-Urinary Diseases

Nephritis, Kidney Diseases, and Pyelonephritis

Atractylodes Combination

Acute nephritis and nephrosis with severe edema

Hoelen Five Herb Formula

Acute nephritis, nephrosis, pyelonephritis with severe thirst; heavy head, edema, vomiting, decreased urinary volume

Minor Blue Dragon Combination

Nephritis, nephrosis following fever; mild edema and decreased urinary volume

Minor Bupleurum Combination with Hoelen Five Herb Formula

Nephritis, nephrosis; thirst, nausea, loss of appetite, albuminuria with slow recovery rate, pyelonephritis, moderate fever, lower back pain. The formula is more effective if given with Hoelen Five Herb Formula.

Polyporus Combination

Pyelonephritis, urethritis, and nephritis; increased frequency in urination, painful or difficult urination with blood.

Ginseng and Tang-kuei Formula

Chronic nephritis, nephrosis from chills, frequent urination but decreased volume. Minor Bupleurum Combination is added when there is a tendency toward albuminura and malaise.

Rehmannia Eight Formula

Chronic nephritis with mild edema, nephrosis, renal atrophy, pyelonephritis, lower back pain, urinary retention, hypertension, nocturia, and increased frequency of urination in the elderly

Bupleurum and Dragon Bone Combination

Chronic nephritis, nephrosis, kidney atrophy; hypertension, constipation, periumbilical palpitation

Persica and Rhubarb Combination

Chronic nephritis, nephrosis, kidney atrophy; headache, flushing, constipation, hypertension

Capillaris Combination with Hoelen Five Herb Formula

Nephritis, nephrosis, liver failure; thirst, chest distress, constipation

Bupleurum and Cinnamon Combination

Nephritis, nephrosis, pyelonephritis with headache, moderate fever, nausea, loss of appetite

Renal and Gall Stones

Polyporus Combination

Difficult or painful urination with bloody urine

Hoelen Five Herb Formula with Minor Bupleurum Combination

Thirst, decreased urinary volume, loss of appetite, lower back pain

Major Zanthoxylum Combination

Severe abdominal pain, tension, vomiting after taking other medication

Rehmannia Eight Formula

Lower back pain and frequent urination with discomfort

Rhubarb and Moutan Combination, Persica and Rhubarb Combination, and Coix Combination

Pain in the lower abdomen, constipation, suppressed urination

Siler and Platycodon Formula

Obesity with constipation

Polyporus Combination

Difficult or painful urination, bloody urine, gonorrheal urethritis

Hoelen Five Herb Formula

Thirst, turbid urine, frequent urination

Rehmannia Eight Formula

Chills in elderly patients; also for postpartum urinary discomfort in women or a swollen prostate in men

Rhubarb and Moutan Combination

Constipation, urinary retention or enlarged prostate, gonorrheal symptoms

Nocturnal Emission, Impotence, and Sexual Neurasthenia

Bupleurum and Dragon Bone Combination

Thoracic distress, palpitation, constipation, severe psychoneurosis

Major Bupleurum Combination

Same symptoms as Bupleurum and Dragon Bone Combination with heart distress, stiff shoulders, tinnitus, and malaise

Siler and Platycodon Formula

Obesity, constipation, a tendency toward impaired health

Rehmannia Eight Formula

Thirst caused by chills and nocturia in climacteric men and women

Cinnamon and Dragon Bone Combination

Symptoms similar to Bupleurum and Dragon Bone Combination but without constipation

Ginseng and Astragalus Combination
Delicate health, a tendency toward extreme fatigue, loss of appetite, night sweats

Eucommia and Rehmannia Formula with Rehmannia Eight Formula
Pale complexion, vertigo and dizziness, lower back pain, aching and weak legs, mental weakness, watery semen, a sinking and small pulse without vigor

Ginseng and Longan Combination, Ginseng Nutritive Combination, and Ginseng and Tang-kuei Ten Combination
A heart and spleen supplement. Chlorotic complexion, loss of appetite, fatigue, weary arms and legs.

Tonic Decoction
Supplements kidneys and stabilizes emotions. Injured kidneys from fright and emotional distress (fright and doubt, palpitations, insomnia).

Gentiana Combination
Downward moist fever; feverish, ruddy urine; yellow, sticky fur on the tongue; a soft, quick pulse

V. Blood Diseases

Anemia, Purpura, and Bleeding

Ginseng and Tang-kuei Formula
Anemia, chills, and decreased volume with increased frequency of urination

Ginseng and Astragalus Combination
Anemia associated with chronic diseases, poor digestion, loss of appetite, tendency to become severely fatigued, night sweats

Bupleurum, Cinnamon, and Ginger Combination
Poor health, anemia, mental instability, insomnia, palpitation, a tendency toward diarrhea

Minor Bupleurum Combination
Childhood anemia and loss of appetite with moderate fever or fatigue

Tang-kuei and Gelatin Combination

Anemia from excessive hemorrhaging and purpura

Bupleurum and Cinnamon Combination

Chronic rheumatoid purpura. Atractylodes Combination is more effective in the primary stage

Blood Disease

Bupleurum and Paeonia Formula

Menopausal disturbances, irregular menses, emotional instability, fatigue, headache, constipation, lumbago

Tang-kuei Four Combination

Blood weakness, gynecological problems, chilblains

Ginseng and Longan Combination

Delicate health with gastrointestinal weakness; bleeding, anemia, amnesia, and neurosis brought on by overwork; irregular menses; loss of appetite after loss of blood

VI. Metabolic Disorders

Hypertrophy

Siler and Platycodon Formula

Good health but a tendency toward constipation and obesity

Major Bupleurum Combination

Heart distress with constipation, stiff shoulders, dizziness, tinnitus, hypertension

Major Bupleurum Combination with Cinnamon and Hoelen Formula

Headache from suppressed or scanty menstruation, occasional flushing, chest distress. If there is severe constipation, Major Bupleurum Combination is prescribed jointly with Persica and Rhubarb Combination.

Stephania and Astragalus Combination
Edema with clear, pale skin; excessive sweating; a propensity to tire easily

Diabetes Mellitus

Rehmannia Eight Formula
Excessive and frequent urination, thirst, fatigue, lower back pain or cold waist, edema, loss of sexual desire

Ginseng and Gypsum Combination
Dry throat, extreme thirst that is more severe than that of Rehmannia Eight Formula but without lower back pain or cold waist

Major Bupleurum Combination with Hoelen Five Herb Formula
Frequent urination with decreased volume, thirst, cardiac distress with constipation

Ophiopogon Combination with platycodon and gypsum
Very poor health with complicating tuberculosis

VII. Diseases of the Endocrine Glands

Goiter in the Young

Ginseng and Tang-kuei Formula
Goiter in young women with anemia and cold extremities

Pinellia and Magnolia Combination
Cardiac hyperfunction, head sweats, insomnia, sore throat, a tendency toward diarrhea in persons of slender build

Bupleurum and Dragon Bone Combination
Excitability, palpitation, insomnia, constipation

VIII. Diseases of the Joints, Muscles, and Tendons

Rheumatism, Arthritis, and Tendonitis

Ma-huang and Coix Combination

Subacute and chronic rheumatism, pain in the joints or tendons, edema and pain in cold weather

Cinnamon, Atractylodes, and Aconite Combination

Chronic rheumatism, tendonitis, stiff shoulders, cold with pain, numbness, impaired motion

Pueraria Combination

Acute rheumatism; tendonitis; pain and stiffness in the shoulders, neck, and back

Ma-huang Combination

For the severe pain of acute rheumatism and tendonitis

Atractylodes Combination

Acute arthritis and rheumatism and severe edema

Stephania and Astragalus Combination

Chronic arthritis; rheumatism; impaired movement; edema with clear, pale skin; mild foot pain

Cinnamon and Hoelen Formula

Arthritis from an injury, hyperemia, swelling, impaired movement

Siler and Platycodon Formula

Obesity, constipation, and arthritis of the shoulders in patients over fifty years old

Rhubarb and Moutan Combination with coix

Tendonitis and constipation

Chin-chiu and Tu-huo Combination, Chianghuo and Turmeric Combination, and Siler Combination

Rheumatism with fever, pain and swelling of the joints

Wu-tou Combination, Wu-tou and Earthworm Formula

Rheumatism without fever; sporadic joint pain which intensifies during cold weather; localized pallor; chills in the affected area

Coix Formula, Alisma and Chianghuo Combination, and Clematis and Stephania Combination

Numbness of skin and muscles, severe swelling of limb joints, deformed joints, pain, muscular atrophy

Cinnamon and Anemarrhena Combination

Fever, mild chills, swelling with burning joint pain during hot weather

IX. Diseases of the Nervous System

Neuralgia and Numbness of the Facial Nerves

Cinnamon, Atractylodes, and Aconite Combination

Chronic neuralgia and numbness of the facial nerves with chills

Pueraria Combination

Acute primary neuralgia and numbness of the facial nerves

Siler and Platycodon Formula

Chronic neuralgia, obesity, a tendency toward constipation

Hoelen Five Herb Formula

Trigeminal neuralgia, thirst, and decreased urinary volume. Usually taken with Pueraria Combination.

Bupleurum and Cinnamon Combination

Intercostal neuralgia and chest distress may respond to Minor Bupleurum Combination. Major Bupleurum Combination is prescribed for persons with severe constipation with hard stools. Bupleurum and Scute Combination is prescribed for soft stools.

Persica and Rhubarb Combination
Sciatic neuralgia, headache, constipation

Tang-kuei, Evodia, and Ginger Combination
Sciatic neuralgia, cold extremities, a tendency toward anemia

Rehmannia Eight Formula
Sciatic neuralgia, chills, diabetes mellitus

Cinnamon and Hoelen Formula
Sciatic neuralgia from difficult menstruation or from trauma

Neurasthenia, Hysteria, and Insomnia

Bupleurum and Dragon Bone Combination
Chest distress with constipation, excitability, palpitation, insomnia without weakness

Coptis and Scute Formula
Flushing reaction, stomach distress, ocular hyperemia, nosebleeds

Pinellia and Magnolia Combination
Melancholia, hysteria, cardiac hyperfunction, distress extending from the throat to the chest

Cyperus and Perilla Formula
More severe melancholia than in Pinellia and Magnolia Combination with headache, insomnia, and loss of appetite

Bupleurum, Cinnamon, and Ginger Combination
Neurasthenia, delicate health, insomnia, asthma, palpitation, head sweats, night sweats, a tendency to pass soft stools—all resulting from hysteria

Ginseng and Astragalus Combination
Hysteria, weak digestion, anorexia

Atractylodes and Hoelen Combination
Headache, insomnia, cardiac hyperfunction with decreased urinary volume, postural vertigo

97

Ginseng and Tang-kuei Formula
Female complaints; chills, headache, psychoneurotic menopausal disorders

X. Pediatrics

Measles, Parotitis, Rickets, Vesicles, Nocturia, Noctiphobia, and Delicate Health

Pueraria Combination
Measles, primary parotitis, headache, high fever, feeling of extreme cold, night-mares.

Minor Bupleurum Combination
Poor health and delayed symptoms of Pueraria Combination with mild fever and loss of appetite

Minor Cinnamon and Paeonia Combination
Nutrient for delicate health, rickets, nocturia, noctiphobia

Atractylodes Combination
Acute herpes simplex with copious secretion; healthy children with enuresis

Bupleurum and Dragon Bone Combination
Noctiphobia and a tendency toward neurasthenia in people with good health and appetite who are constipated

Cinnamon and Dragon Bone Combination
Noctiphobia, nocturia, impaired health resulting from psychoneurosis

XI. Surgery

Editor's Note: Chinese medicine does not employ surgery itself, it being a Western treatment. However, traditionally the following conditions are listed under surgery because they usually involve lancing.

Burns, Frostbite, Furuncle, Anal and Bone Ulcers, Lymphadenitis, Scrofula, and Intestinal Disorders

Cinnamon and Hoelen Formula

First degree frostbite, chills, darkened complexion

Persica and Rhubarb Combination

Same symptoms as Cinnamon and Hoelen Formula with constipation

Ginseng and Tang-kuei Formula

Frostbite, cold arms and legs, a tendency toward anemia; also prevents frostbite

Pinellia and Ginger Combination

Third degree frostbite; same symptoms as Ginseng and Tang-kuei Formula but a chronic condition

Pueraria Combination

Primary furunculosis and anthrax with inflammation, fever, and coldness. Platycodon and gypsum are added to the formula for suppuration.

Bupleurum and Schizonepeta Formula

Furuncles, anthrax, lymphadenitis, perianal ulcer, lingering diseases or chronic inflammation, fever, suppuration

Eriocheir and Viper Formula

Furuncles, anthrax, anal and osseous ulcers, scrofula, inflammation, and local suppuration. This formula is not recommended for primary or subacute inflammation in severe conditons.

Major Bupleurum Combination

Furuncles, anthrax, heart distress with severe constipation

Siler and Platycodon Formula

Furuncles, anthrax, obesity with constipation

Rhubarb and Moutan Combination with coix

Furuncles and anthrax; constipation caused by disorders of the lower body

Minor Bupleurum Combination with platycodon and gypsum
    Lymphadenitis, scrofula, moderate fever or chills, loss of appetite

Ginseng and Astragalus Combination with Eriocheir and Viper Formula
    Osseous ulcers, delicate health, fatigue, malaise, loss of appetite

Major Zanthoxylum Combination
    Rectal prolapse, severe abdominal pain, acute vomiting.

Minor Cinnamon and Paeonia Combination
    Rectal prolapse, symptoms more moderate than for Major Zanthoxylum Combination with no vomiting and a tendency toward psychoneurosis

Lithospermum Ointment
    Applied externally on burns, frostbite, furuncles, anthrax, and anal ulcers

XII. Anal Disorders

Hemorrhoids and Rectal Prolapse

Cimicifuga Combination
    Hemorrhoids, rectal prolapse, constipation with slight bleeding, local pain, itching

Ginseng and Tang-kuei Formula
    Hemorrhoids, rectal prolapse, chills with constipation, severe diarrhea after taking Tang-kuei and Bupleurum Combination

Major Bupleurum Combination
    Hemorrhoids, rectal prolapse, heart distress with constipation, anal fissures

Cinnamon and Hoelen Formula
    Hemorrhoids, flushing, hemorrhage without a propensity toward anemia

Persica and Rhubarb Combination
    Hemorrhoids with severe, dark red bleeding and serious constipation

Tang-kuei and Gelatin Combination
    Hemorrhoidal bleeding; anemia from excessive hemorrhage

Ginseng and Astragalus Combination

Rectal prolapse, fatigue, loss of appetite, slow recovery because of delicate health.

Eriocheir and Viper Formula

Hemorrhoids with continuous watery suppuration and delayed granulation

Lithospermum Ointment

Applied externally on hemorrhoids

XIII. Obstetrical Problems

Habitual Abortion, Nephritis in Pregnancy, Delayed Bleeding, Mastitis, Childbirth Fever, Postpartum Beriberi, and Pain

Pinellia and Magnolia Combination

Nausea, throat discomfort, psychoneurosis

Pinellia Combination

Severe nausea, loss of appetite, a tendency toward soft stools

Ginseng and Tang-kuei Formula with Minor Bupleurum Combination

Habitual abortion; prevention of nephritis during pregnancy; mild pain after overexertion. The formula should be taken by pregnant women to promote fast recovery of health during the postpartum period and to lessen chances of childbirth fever, loss of appetite, and chills.

Pueraria Combination with platycodon and gypsum

Mastitis, fever, chills, stiff shoulders

Minor Bupleurum Combination with platycodon and gypsum

Mastitis, fever, chills, tongue fur, dry lips, thirst, loss of appetite

Bupleurum and Schizonepeta Formula

Mastitis and susceptibility to suppuration

Cinnamon and Hoelen Formula

Successive bleeding after aborting

Tang-kuei and Gelatin Combination

Hemorrhage during pregnancy, delayed bleeding, a tendency toward anemia

Rehmannia Eight Formula

Beriberi following childbirth; thirst and cold, numb arms and legs

XIV. Gynecological Problems

Menstrual Disorders, Vicarious Menstruation, Congenital Anomalies, Retroverted and Prolapsed Uterus, Endometritis, Uterine Swelling, Oophoritis, Salpingitis, Sterility, and Menopausal Disorders

Ginseng and Tang-kuei Formula

Cold conformation with malaise, vertigo, heavy headedness, frequent urination, and delicate health; menstrual and menopausal disorders, vicarious menstruation, congenital anomalies, retroverted and prolapsed uterus, uterine bleeding,
spontaneous abortion, interrupted pregnancy, postpartum weakness, kidney
infections during pregnancy, postpartum beriberi, pallor from anemia, chills
with headache, dizziness, palpitation, stiff shoulders, abdominal pain, fatigue,
thirst, polyuria, leukorrhea

Cinnamon and Hoelen Formula

Headache; flushing; lower abdominal pain; discoloration of the face, lips, or gums
("old blood") with cold arms and legs; a tendency to hemorrhage in the head
area and tinnitus with no anemia; difficult and vicarious menstruation; absent
or suppressed menses; leukorrhea; endometritis; uterine swelling; retroverted
uterus; inflamed ovary or fallopian tube; sterility; menopausal disorders; uterine
bleeding

Persica and Rhubarb Combination

Constipation, headache, cold arms and legs, and associated symptoms of Cinnamon and Hoelen Formula

Rhubarb and Moutan Combination

Constipation and lower right abdominal pain associated with symptoms of Persica
and Rhubarb Combination without headache or chills

Tang-kuei and Gelatin Combination

Menorrhagia or delayed menstruation, uterine bleeding, bleeding hemorrhoids

Pinellia and Magnolia Combination

Suppressed or scanty menstruation from temporary psychoneurosis

Cyperus and Perilla Formula

Suppressed or scanty menstruation from psychoneurosis; menopausal disorders; melancholia and loss of appetite

Atractylodes and Hoelen Combination

Menstrual irregularities and disorders, ocular hyperemia, headache, dizziness, occasional anemia. When Ginseng and Tang-kuei Formula and Cinnamon and Hoelen Formula have not been effective, this formula is used.

Coptis and Scute Formula

Menorrhagia, vicarious menstruation, mild constipation with soft stools

Coptis and Rhubarb Combination

Menorrhagia, vicarious menstruation, severe flushing, chronic constipation

Pinellia and Magnolia Combination

Psychosomatic digestive disorders (throat and chest distress, nausea, and vomiting); hysteria; menopausal disorders; morning sickness

Minor Bupleurum Combination

Loss of appetite; malaise; thoracic distress; functional disorders of the stomach, intestines, and liver. The formula is commonly used in conjunction with Tang-kuei and Paeonia Formula, Cinnamon and Hoelen Formula, and Pinellia and Magnolia Combination for improving general health and nutrition.

Tang-kuei and Paeonia Combination

Irregular menses, habitual miscarriage, stagnant blood in weak patients

XV. Skin Diseases

**Dermatitis or Eczema, Urticaria or Hives, Maculae, Vesicles,
Athlete's Foot, Warts, Ringworm or Fungus, Baldness,
and Infected Suppurative Crusts**

Bupleurum and Schizonepeta Formula

Eczema, urticaria or hives, infected suppurative crusts, ringworm, dermato-
phytosis—all chronic and with slight secretion

Tang-kuei and Arctium Formula

Chronic eczema and hives

Pueraria Combination

Eczema and infected crusts with primary fever and severe itching

Atractylodes Combination

Eczema, infected crusts, and ringworm—all with acute vesicles or copious secretion

Cinnamon and Hoelen Formula with Minor Bupleurum Combination

Eczema, hives, facial vesicles, ringworm, athlete's foot, or maculae; chills, loss
of appetite, occasional constipation

Persica and Rhubarb Combination

Local dark color along with symptoms of Cinnamon and Hoelen Formula with
Minor Bupleurum Combination plus chills, headache, constipation, pain in the
lower abdomen

Rhubarb and Moutan Combination

The same symptoms as Persica and Rhubarb Combination with constipation
but without headache or chills

Rehmannia Eight Formula

Eczema or hives and glycosuria in the elderly with coldness or delicate health
and with thirst and irregular urination

Capillaris Combination

Hives, thirst, chest distress, constipation. The combination is taken with Hoelen Five Herb Formula if the condition is chronic. Improves liver function and relieves constipation.

Cinnamon Combination with Ma-huang Combination

Hives, flushing with moderate fever, severe itching

Major Bupleurum Combination

Eczema, hives or facial vesicles with balding, heart distress and constipation, a tendency towards liver failure; stiff shoulder; tinnitus

Siler and Platycodon Formula

Eczema, hives, rosacea, athlete's foot, balding, obesity with constipation

Ginseng and Tang-kuei Formula

Maculae, athlete's foot, warts, ringworm, anemia with chills, increased urinary frequency but decreased volume. The formula is used with Coix Combination for dry skin.

Bupleurum and Dragon Bone Combination

Balding, periumbilical palpitation, mental instability, constipation

Cinnamon and Dragon Bone Combination

Falling hair, psychoneurosis with fatigue, waning sexual desire; no constipation

Ma-huang and Coix Combination

Various types of warts. If the warts are severe, Coix Combination should be used concurrently.

Coix Combination

Various types of warts, papules, and skin eruptions. Treatment may continue for one or two months.

Eriocheir and Viper Formula with Coix Combination

Suppurative dermatosis. These formulas are not given if the patient has an acute or subacute febrile illness, a reddish color, or severe pain.

Lithospermum Ointment

Applied externally on facial vesicles, infected crusts, athlete's foot

XVI. Ophthalmology

Sty, Dacryocystitis, Conjunctivitis, Keratitis, Trachoma, Ocular Eczema, Iritis, Cataract, Glaucoma, Nyctalopia, and Ocular Bleeding

Pueraria Combination

Primary ocular hyperemia with tearing or exudate, headache, stiff shoulders

Minor Blue Dragon Combination

Acute or subacute ocular hyperemia, excessive tearing

Atractylodes Combination

Acute orbital swelling and considerable tearing

Atractylodes and Hoelen Combination

Chronic ocular hyperemia, tearing, dizziness

Hoelen Five Herb Formula

Abundant tearing, thirst, fatigue

Minor Bupleurum Combination

Malaise and loss of appetite

Ginseng and Tang-kuei Formula

Eye ailments in women with chills, anemia, menstrual irregularity, and post-partum illness

Cinnamon and Hoelen Formula

Female complaints with chills, flushing, and chronic ocular hyperemia

Persica and Rhubarb Combination

The same symptoms as Cinnamon and Hoelen Formula plus severe constipation

Siler and Platycodon Formula

Obesity with constipation

Bupleurum and Dragon Bone Combination
   Marked psychoneurosis, palpitation, insomnia, constipation

Bupleurum and Schizonepeta Formula
   Suppuration

Eriocheir and Viper Formula
   Chronic and delayed suppuration

Minor Cinnamon and Paeonia Combination
   Delicate health and recurrent illness

Rehmannia Eight Formula
   Symptoms associated with diabetes mellitus due to dietary deficiency or old age

Coptis and Rhubarb Combination
   Flushing with hyperemia and stomach distress with constipation

Coptis and Rhubarb Combination with Coptis and Scute Formula
   Similar symptoms to Coptis and Rhubarb Combination but diarrhea occurs after taking Coptis and Rhubarb Combination alone

XVII. Ear, Nose, and Throat Diseases

Otitis Externa, Otitis Media, Rhinitis, Tonsillitis, Laryngitis, Pharyngitis, and Suppuration

Pueraria Combination
   Pain in initial stages, alternate chills and fever, headache, nasal congestion, chronic suppuration, stiff shoulders. For suppuration, add platycodon and gypsum.

Minor Bupleurum Combination with platycodon and gypsum
   Chronic loss of appetite

Major Bupleurum Combination
   Delayed constipation, tinnitus, stiff shoulders

Bupleurum and Schizonepeta Formula

Suppurative otitis externa, otitis media, nasal congestion with dense exudate

Minor Blue Dragon Combination

Nasal congestion with copious thin secretion

Atractylodes and Hoelen Combination

Chronic nasal congestion, suppuration, dizziness

Pinellia and Magnolia Combination

Tonsillitis, pharyngitis, laryngitis, hoarseness or loss of voice

Minor Cinnamon and Paeonia Combination

Enlarged tonsils; chronically impaired health in children with recurrent illness

Eriocheir and Viper Formula

Otitis media with suppuration and chronic discharge. The formula is usually given with other prescriptions.

XVIII. Dental Problems

Caries, Periodontitis, and Alveolar Suppuration

Pueraria Combination

Dental caries, periodontitis, pyorrhea, primary-stage fever, headache, stiff shoulders, severe pain. Platycodon and gypsum are added for suppuration.

Persica and Rhubarb Combination

Periodontitis, alveolar pyorrhea, chills, flushing, constipation, purpuric gingival abscess, chronic pain

Major Bupleurum Combination with Siler and Platycodon Formula

Alveolar pyorrhea and cardiac distress with constipation. Obese patients require Siler and Platycodon Formula.

Coptis and Scute Formula

Alveolar pyorrhea and bleeding gums

Ginseng and Astragalus Combination

Alveolar pyorrhea, delicate health with loss of appetite, a tendency toward anemia, slow recovery periods

Rehmannia Eight Formula

Alveolar pyorrhea and symptoms associated with diabetes mellitus

Eriocheir and Viper Formula

Alveolar pyorrhea and continuous thick suppuration which does not respond to chemotherapy

XIX. *Ch'i* Disease

Major Four Herb Combination, Major Six Herb Combination, and Ginseng and Astragalus Combination

Ch'i weakness; shortness of breath; sweating; vertigo; palpitations; disinclination to talk; moist, white tongue; sinking, slow, feeble pulse

Pinellia and Magnolia Combination

Stagnant *ch'i*, sensation of a lump in the throat or abdomen, nervousness

Minor Pinellia and Hoelen Combination

Uprushing *ch'i*, coughing, vomiting, dry heaves, headache, vertigo

Cinnamon and Pinellia Combination

Sensation of *ch'i* rising in chest and throat, irritability

XX. Water Disease

Hoelen Five Herb Formula

Thirst, headache, nausea, vomiting, intoxication

Polyporus Combination

Dysuria, hematuria, cystitis, urethritis, urinary stones

Hoelen and Alisma Combination

Dyspnea, edema, ascites, peritonitis, cirrhosis. Strong patients only.

Hoelen, Alisma, and Ginger Combination with Atractylodes and Hoelen Combination

Headache, dizziness, stomach distention and pain, vomiting, palpitation

Hoelen and Schizandra Combination

Asthma, wheezing, chronic bronchitis, emphysema. Especially in old and weak persons.

Hoelen, Licorice, and Schizandra Combination

Cough, palpitation, cold feet and hands, paralysis, kidney weakness

Ginseng and Ginger Combination

Stomach distention, gastroptosis, peptic ulcer. Very weak patients only.

Hoelen, Licorice, and Jujube Combination

Mixed *ch'i* and water disease symptoms, headache, sweating, vomiting, dizziness, palpitation, uprushing *ch'i*

Hoelen and Ginger Combination

Sensation of "sitting in water" (an extreme bloated feeling in the lower torso); heavy, cold legs; edema

Hoelen and Licorice Combination

Sweating without thirst, insomnia, headache, palpitations, cold extremities, dry heaves

Major Blue Dragon Combination

Pneumonia, conjunctivitis, rheumatism, acute tuberculosis. Strong patients only.

Minor Blue Dragon Combination

Cough, wheezing, eczema, edema, urticaria

Ma-huang Combination

Asthma, aching body without perspiration, wheezing

Ma-huang and Atractylodes Combination

Cough, body pain without perspiration, edema

Ma-huang and Coix Combination

Rheumatic pain, arthritis, edema

Part 2: Preferred Medication for Symptomatic Treatment

I. Fever

Ma-huang Combination

Acute fever with chills, headache, joint and muscular pain, but without sweating

Pueraria Combination

Stiff back or shoulders along with symptoms of Ma-huang Combination, but less severe body pain

Minor Blue Dragon Combination

Same symptoms as Pueraria Combination with difficult breathing, severe cough, and thirst, or with excessive sputum

Minor Bupleurum Combination

Thoracic or abdominal distress with or without sensation of pressure, chronic moderate fever, white tongue coating, loss of appetite

Major Bupleurum Combination

Same symptoms as Minor Bupleurum Combination along with stomach distress and rigidity, yellow or white tongue discoloration, severe constipation

Bupleurum and Cinnamon Combination

Moderate fever, night sweats, headache, chest pain, loss of appetite

Bupleurum, Cinnamon, and Ginger Combination

Impaired health with moderate fever, thirst, night sweats, heavy head, anorexia, diarrhea or soft stools, sensation of palpitation in the chest and abdomen

Bupleurum and Dragon Bone Combination

Neurosis, mental instability, insomnia, sensation of periumbilical palpitation, constipation, moderate fever

Bupleurum and Scute Combination

Moderate fever, chest and back pain, pulmonary edema, cough, chronic expectoration

Ginseng Nutritive Combination

Poor health causing chronic cough and moderate or severe fever with heavy head, fatigue, and loss of appetite

Ginseng and Astragalus Combination

Convalescence or delicate health with marked fatigue, moderate or severe fever with heavy head, fatigue, loss of appetite, and anemia

Cinnamon and Dragon Bone Combination

Debilitation or psychoneurosis, tendency to sweat, cardiac hyperfunction, and sensation of palpitation over the lower abdomen

Minor Cinnamon and Paeonia Combination

Weakness, lack of vigor, fatigue, palpitation and thirst with or without abdominal pain and moderate fever

Cyperus and Perilla Formula

Psychoneurosis and delicate health with headache, heavy head, moderate fever, and loss of appetite

Ginseng and Gypsum Combination

Sensation of warmth or fever, thirst, polyuria, sugar in the urine

Hoelen Five Herb Formula

Moderate fever or feeling of warmth, thirst, inability to urinate, diarrhea

Rehmannia Eight Formula

Thirst, polyuria, lower back pain, sensation of warmth in the feet and waist

Ophiopogon Combination

Sudden severe cough, sore throat or warm flushing sensation from the throat to the chest, thirst

II. Headache and Flushing Sensation

Ma-huang Combination

Fever with headache and active joint and muscular pain

Pueraria Combination

Fever, frontal headache or migraine, acute shoulder stiffness

Pueraria Combination with platycodon and gypsum

Dense nasal exudate, stuffy nose, headache, stiff shoulders, inflammation of the ear with purulent discharge

Coptis and Rhubarb Combination

Severe constipation, stomach distress, flushing, mental instability, or insomnia

Major Bupleurum Combination

Severe constipation, cardiac distress, insomnia, headache

Cinnamon and Hoelen Formula

Headache, flushing, nosebleeds, cold feet and waist, lower back pain, abdominal pain, painful or difficult menstruation

Persica and Rhubarb Combination

Severe symptoms of Cinnamon and Hoelen Formula with constipation and dark red lips or fingers

Atractylodes and Hoelen Combination

A tendency toward anemia with headache, dizziness, and palpitation

Minor Bupleurum Combination

Moderate fever, malaise, loss of appetite, mild headache

Bupleurum and Cinnamon Combination

Moderate fever, night sweats, headache, heavy head, abdominal and chest pain

Cyperus and Perilla Formula

Severe psychoneurosis, headache, and anorexia in delicate females and elderly males

Cinnamon, Atractylodes, and Aconite Combination

Cold lower body, a propensity toward flushing, speech disorders, with or without numb arms and legs

III. Heaviness of the Head and Dizziness

Atractylodes and Hoelen Combination

A tendency toward anemia, headache, dizziness, palpitation

Ginseng and Tang-kuei Formula

Anemia with cold feet and waist, frequent urination with decreased volume, heavy head, vertigo. If a cold stomach follows the use of the formula, Magnolia and Ginger Formula should be given. If loss of appetite occurs, the patient should take Minor Bupleurum Combination.

Tang-kuei and Gelatin Combination

Excessive hemorrhage, anemia, heavy head, dizziness

Minor Bupleurum Combination with Hoelen Five Herb Formula

Moderate fever, thirst, propensity to tire easily, heavy head, decreased urine

Vitality Combination

Severely cold arms and legs, weak digestion, palpitation, dizziness, diarrhea or soft stools

Pinellia and Magnolia Combination with Minor Bupleurum Combination

Psychoneurosis, odd sensation in the chest or throat, loss of appetite, malaise, heavy head

Hoelen Combination

Stomach distention, palpitation, loss of appetite, vertigo

Bupleurum, Cinnamon, and Ginger Combination

Poor health with moderate fever, night sweats, headache, and anorexia

Ginseng Nutritive Combination

Chronic cough, fever, heavy head, and loss of appetite—all associated with poor health

Bupleurum and Cinnamon Combination

Moderate fever, night sweats, heavy head, chest or abdominal pain

IV. Palpitation and Cardiac Hyperfunction

Bupleurum and Dragon Bone Combination

Mental instability or insomnia and constipation, periumbilical palpitation

Bupleurum, Cinnamon, and Ginger Combination

Loss of appetite from invalidism, cardiac hyperfunction, periumbilical palpitation, a tendency toward dry mouth or lips

Pinellia and Magnolia Combination with Cinnamon and Dragon Bone Combination

Delicate health from psychoneurosis; cardiac hyperfunction or lower abdominal palpitation; a tendency to sweat

Ginseng and Tang-kuei Formula

Anemia with cold feet and waist, abdominal pain, dizziness, palpitation, stiff shoulders

Atractylodes and Hoelen Combination

A tendency toward anemia, headache, palpitation, vertigo

Hoelen Combination

Abdominal distention, palpitation, nausea or anorexia

Minor Cinnamon and Paeonia Combination

Infirmity, palpitation, fatigue, abdominal pain

Stephania and Ginseng Combination

Distressed stomach with palpitation, difficult breathing, slight cough, thirst, edema

Vitality Combination

Cold arms and legs, heavy head, palpitation, decreased urine, diarrhea

V. Dry Throat and Lips

Ginseng and Gypsum Combination
>   Thirst, frequent and excessive urination

Hoelen Five Herb Formula
>   Thirst, decreased urine with abdominal pain or edema, diarrhea

Rehmannia Eight Formula
>   Thirst, excessive urination, cold waist with or without lower back pain, sensation of urinary retention

Capillaris Combination with Hoelen Five Herb Formula
>   Thirst, decreased urinary volume with turbidity, constipation and distressed chest

Polyporus Combination
>   Difficult or painful urination and urinary retention, thirst, excessive urination. If the lower body feels cold, Ginseng and Tang-kuei Formula should be given.

Atractylodes Combination
>   Severe edema, decreased urinary volume, difficult breathing, acute joint pain

Ma-huang and Apricot Combination
>   Severe cough, difficult breathing, thirst, a tendency to sweat

Minor Bupleurum Combination with Hoelen Five Herb Formula
>   White-coated tongue, bitter taste in the mouth, loss of appetite, fatigue, thirst

Atractylodes and Hoelen Combination with Minor Bupleurum Combination
>   Headache, heavy head, dizziness, palpitation, anorexia, decreased urinary volume, occasional thirst

Bupleurum, Cinnamon, and Ginger Combination
>   Delicate health with moderate fever, loss of appetite, night sweats, asthma, thirst, a tendency towards soft stools

Ophiopogon Combination

Poor health with a tendency toward flushing or sensation of fever, thirst, severe cough, and pharyngeal pain

Minor Cinnamon and Paeonia Combination

Impaired health, loss of vigor, fatigue, palpitation, abdominal pain or thirst

Stephania and Ginseng Combination

Severe difficulty breathing, cough, edema, sweating, thirst

Vitality Combination

Severe chills, dry throat but without desire to drink liquids, chronic diarrhea or soft stools

VI. Diseases of the Mouth

Coptis and Scute Formula

Stomach distress, decreased stool volume, a rough feeling inside the mouth, flushing, a tendency to hemorrhage

Capillaris Combination

Coarse or dry feeling in the throat and on the lips, constipation, chest distress, decreased urinary volume

Pinellia Combination

Stomach distress, abdominal pain with gas, coarse feeling in mouth, diarrhea or soft stools

Bupleurum, Cinnamon, and Ginger Combination

Delicate health with moderate fever, head sweats or night sweats, dry or rough lips

VII. Stiff Shoulders or Neck

Pueraria Combination

Chills with stiff neck, shoulders, or back or joint pain; with or without fever

Minor Bupleurum Combination

Tendency toward fatigue, loss of appetite with peculiar mouth odor, stiff shoulders or neck. If the symptoms are marked and associated with severe constipation, Major Bupleurum Combination should be prescribed.

Cinnamon and Hoelen Formula

Headache, flushing, tinnitus, stiff shoulders, cold waist and feet. If the symptoms are marked and associated with severe constipation, the patient should take Minor Bupleurum Combination.

Siler and Platycodon Formula

Obesity with headache, stiff shoulders, chest distress, and constipation

Ginseng and Tang-kuei Formula

Anemia, chills, heavy head, stiff shoulders, abdominal pain, lower back pain

Cyperus and Perilla Formula

Psychoneurosis, headache, or stiff shoulders in the elderly or women with delicate health

VIII. Chest or Back Pain

Bupleurum and Cinnamon Combination

Severe stomach or chest pain and nausea

Bupleurum and Scute Combination

Chest pain, chronic expectoration, stomach distress, occasional back pain

Major Bupleurum Combination

Cardiac distress and chest pain, pressure in the chest and abdomen with severe constipation. If there is thirst and decreased urinary volume, the patient should take Hoelen Five Herb Formula

Minor Blue Dragon Combination

Chest pain, difficult breathing, cough with frothy sputum

Minor Bupleurum Combination

Chest or abdominal distress, pressure, stiff shoulders, or back pain

Bupleurum and Dragon Bone Combination
Mental instability or insomnia with constipation, periumbilical palpitation, mild chest pain

Ophiopogon Combination
Severe cough, flushing, chest pain, thick sputum

Minor Cinnamon and Paeonia Combination
Delicate health, malaise, mild pain and weakness in the back

Rehmannia Eight Formula or Rehmannia Six Formula plus eucommia, lycium fruit, and morinda
Kidney weakness causing lower back pain or chronic pain at waist and knees in the elderly

Tang-kuei Four Combination with persica and carthamus
Low back pain caused by stagnant blood

Bupleurum and Chih-shih Formula with gardenia, paeonia, *tang-kuei,* and raw rehmannia
Sudden chills and fever during menstruation or after childbirth, chest distention, irritability, somatic pain

Pueraria Combination
Stiff neck, severe chills, anhidrosis, a floating and tight pulse

Chih-shih and Arisaema Combination
Stagnant liquid in stomach, pain in shoulders and back, aching and weak hands and arms

Atractylodes and Hoelen Combination plus Chih-shih and Arisaema Combination or Minor Pinellia Combination
Stagnant liquid in stomach, pain in shoulders and back, aching and weak hands and arms, chills in shoulders and back, or chills and pain in either the stomach or the opposing section of the back

Ginseng and Astragalus Combination with *chianghuo* and siler
Backache caused by weak blood vessels overexertion, prolonged sitting

Major Siler Combination
.Pain and swelling in one or both knees

Tang-kuei Four Combination with chaenomeles and coix
Muscular atrophy, difficulty bending or stretching at the articular joints, fever in the palms or feet, a reddish tongue, a small and rapid pulse, an underdeveloped body

G.H.A. and Licorice Combination
Slight pain below the waist, bloating due to edema. Drying agent for wet toxin in the lower warmer.

Astragalus Five Combination with ginseng, eucommia, and cynomorium
Low back pain, impaired kidney *ch'i* from long term overexertion

Ma-huang Combination
Severe chills, anhidrosis, stuffy nose, sniffles, somatic pain, a floating and tight pulse

Cinnamon Combination with ginseng and paeonia
Somatic pain, a sinking and late pulse, impaired flow of yin due to sweating and malnourishment

Gypsum Combination with scute and forsythia
Internal fever or fever of the heart and lungs with perspiration but no reduction of fever, snoring, lethargy, a feeling of heaviness, somatic pain

Ginseng and Astragalus Combination
Heaviness of the limbs and somatic pain from descending yang

Astragalus and Atractylodes Combination
Heaviness of the limbs and somatic pain from descending yang but with weak *ch'i* and slow movements

IX. Nausea and Vomiting

Pinellia and Magnolia Combination

Psychoneurosis with pharmngeal and thoracic distress, nausea, and vomiting. If there is malaise and anorexia, Minor Bupleurum Combination should be added.

Pinellia Combination

Nausea or vomiting, stomach distress with a tendency towards diarrhea or soft stools

Bupleurum and Cinnamon Combination

Chest and severe stomach pain, nausea,·or vomiting

Major Bupleurum Combination

Distress in the chest, abdomen, or heart; nausea or vomiting; severe constipation

Minor Bupleurum Combination

Chest or abdominal distress with nausea or vomiting and loss of appetite

Hoelen Five Herb Formula

Thirst, decreased urinary volume with nausea, vomiting, and abdominal pain

Hoelen Combination

Stomach distention, nausea or vomiting, anorexia, occasional diarrhea

Cardamon and Fennel Formula

Psychoneurosis with stomach pain, chest distress, nausea, and chills

Major Zanthoxylum Combination

Cold abdomen, abdominal distention with pain or nausea, general chills

Vitality Combination

Cold arms and legs, palpitation, dizziness, a tendency toward diarrhea, slight nausea

Stephania and Ginseng Combination

Severe difficulty breathing, cough, stridor, occasional edema, nausea

X. Chills

Cinnamon, Atractylodes, and Aconite Combination

Chills in the lower part of the body, numbness in the arms and legs, disturbed speech, decreased urinary volume, sweating, or a tendency to flush

Rehmannia Eight Formula

Thirst, cold waist and feet, lower back pain, polyuria, and a sensation of urinary retention particularly among elderly people

Major Zanthoxylum Combination

Cold and swollen sensation in the abdomen, abdominal pain, occasional nausea, constipation

Ginseng and Tang-kuei Formula

Anemia with cold waist or feet, decreased urinary volume, polyuria, heaviness of the head, stiff shoulders, dizziness, palpitation, and lower back pain (especially in middle-aged women)

Tang-kuei, Evodia, and Ginger Combination

Same symptoms as Ginseng and Tang-kuei Formula with cold arms, legs, and waist, abdominal distention, cramps from the waist to the feet, and sometimes circulatory disturbances in the peripheral vessels

Tang-kuei and Gelatin Combination

Anemia from excessive hemorrhage, heavy head, vertigo, abdominal pain, lower back pain, general chills

Stephania and Astragalus Combination

"Clean, white" skin, edema, a tendency to tire easily, sweating, swollen feet, chills

Stephania and Ginseng Combination

Stomach distress, difficult breathing, palpitation, cough or stridor, chills

Minor Cinnamon and Paeonia Combination

Delicate health with loss of vigor, fatigue, palpitation, thirst, abdominal pain or distention, chills

Tang-kuei and Paeonia Formula

A delicate body, a tendency toward anemia, headache, asthma, polyuria, chills with moderate abdominal pain

Atractylodes and Hoelen Combination with dry ginger

Chills, heavy feeling at the waist, frequent urination, urinary retention in a chilled body

Cinnamon and Hoelen Formula

Menstrual irregularity, lumbago, stiff shoulders, chills in the arms and legs

Bupleurum, Cinnamon, and Ginger Combination

Weakness with moderate fever, night sweats, thirst, loss of appetite, diarrhea or soft stools, and general chills

Ginseng and Astragalus Combination

Weak digestion or anemia following an illness, malaise, loss of appetite with soft stools, chills

Ginseng Nutritive Combination

Severe cough lingering after an illness, heavy head, loss of appetite, chills

Persica and Rhubarb Combination

Headache, flushing, stiff shoulders, cold feet and waist, lower back pain, pain when pressed on the abdomen, menstrual irregularity, severe constipation

Cinnamon and Hoelen Formula

Moderate symptoms of Persica and Rhubarb Combination but without constipation. Especially for adolescents and unmarried females.

XI. Abdominal Pain

1. General

Minor Cinnamon and Paeonia Combination

Poor health and a tendency to tire easily, abdominal pain, palpitation in the lower abdomen

Major Zanthoxylum Combination

Abdominal chills, pain, and distention, constipation or diarrhea

Vitality Combination

Severely cold arms and legs, heavy head, gas, decreased urinary volume, diarrhea, and abdominal pain

2. Upper Abdomen

Major Bupleurum Combination

Cardiac distress, pressure in the chest or abdomen with severe constipation, nausea, vomiting, and pain in the upper abdomen

Bupleurum and Cinnamon Combination

Severe pain and distress extending from the stomach to the abdomen, and abdominal tension with moderate fever or nausea

Minor Bupleurum Combination

Thoracic or abdominal distress or pain, a white-coated tongue, loss of appetite, nausea, fatigability

Cardamon and Fennel Formula

Psychoneurosis, chest distress, nausea, moderate pain in the abdomen, chills

Magnolia and Ginger Formula

Abdominal distress with distention, diarrhea after meals, abdominal pain before defecation

Bupleurum, Cinnamon, and Ginger Combination

Weakness with moderate fever, dry mouth or lips, loss of appetite, diarrhea or soft stools or abdominal pain

3. Lower Abdomen

Rhubarb and Moutan Combination

Constipation and pain in the lower right abdomen

Persica and Rhubarb Combination

Flushing with headache, stiff shoulders, chills in the lower body, constipation, and lower back or abdominal pain

Cinnamon and Hoelen Formula

Moderate symptoms of Persica and Rhubarb Combination without constipation

Pueraria Combination

Fever; chills; stiff neck, shoulders, or back; abdominal pain; diarrhea and bloody stools. Also for acute symptoms with high fever.

Ginseng and Tang-kuei Formula

Absence of flushing but with heavy head and chills, especially in the feet and waist, and frequent urination with decreased volume and abdominal pain

Tang-kuei, Evodia, and Ginger Combination

Symptoms of Ginseng and Tang-kuei Formula along with abdominal distention, lower back pain or cramps extending from the waist to the feet, a tendency toward chilblains

Tang-kuei and Gelatin Combination

Uterine or hemorrhoidal bleeding with chills and abdominal pain

Pinellia Combination

Stomach distress, nausea or vomiting, loss of appetite, diarrhea, abdominal pain

Cinnamon and Dragon Bone Combination

Lower abdominal tension, sensation of palpitation, abdominal distention or pain

XII. Diarrhea and Soft Stools

Pueraria Combination

Acute diarrhea with fever, chills, and frequent defecation with a feeling of retention

125

Hoelen Five Herb Formula

Thirst, decreased urinary volume, moderate abdominal pain with acute watery diarrhea

Magnolia and Ginger Formula

Stomach distress with diarrhea after meals

Major Bupleurum Combination

Good health, cardiac distress with constipation, diarrhea

Pinellia Combination

Stomach distress, nausea, vomiting or gas, soft stools, diarrhea alternating with constipation

Bupleurum and Cinnamon Combination

Lower back pain or abdominal pain, lower abdominal tension, diarrhea which may be mucoid

Coptis and Scute Formula

Flushing with stomach distress and scanty and occasional soft stools or diarrhea

Bupleurum, Cinnamon, and Ginger Combination

Weakness with moderate fever, loss of appetite, night sweats, dry mouth or lips, and soft stools

Ginseng Nutritive Combination

Loss of appetite and soft stools, delicate health, chronic cough or successive moderate fever

Ginseng and Astragalus Combination

Post illness or impaired digestion, malaise, loss of appetite, soft stools

Hoelen Combination

Distressed and swollen stomach, decreased urine, loss of appetite, frequent diarrhea

Ginseng and Tang-kuei Formula

Chills (especially of the feet and waist), increased frequency of urination with decreased volume, diarrhea or soft stools

Minor Cinnamon and Paeonia Combination

Impaired health, a tendency to tire easily, urinary frequency, abdominal pain, diarrhea

Major Zanthoxylum Combination

Chills in the abdomen; abdominal pain and distention or diarrhea caused by hyperperistalsis

Vitality Combination

Severely cold feet and waist, decreased urinary volume, gas, diarrhea or chronically soft stools

XIII. Constipation

Rhubarb and Moutan Combination

Pain in the lower abdomen, constipation, dark red lips or fingertips

Persica and Rhubarb Combination

Headache, stiff shoulders, tinnitus, chills in the lower body, and symptoms of Rhubarb and Moutan Combination

Major Bupleurum Combination

Cardiac distress, sensation of pressure, severe constipation

Coptis and Rhubarb Combination

Flushing, mental instability with stomach distress and constipation with hard stools. If not effective, add more rhubarb.

Hoelen Five Herb Formula

Distressed chest with thirst, constipation, turbid urine

Bupleurum and Dragon Bone Combination

Severe symptoms of psychoneurosis, insomnia, thoracic distress, and constipation

Siler and Platycodon Formula

Obesity with constipation and occasional stiff shoulders, or thoracic distress

Cinnamon and Hoelen Formula with Major Rhubarb Combination and Coptis and Rhubarb Combination

Flushing with headache, stiff shoulders, difficult menstruation, and constipation

Coptis and Scute Formula

Flushing with stiff neck or shoulders, stomach distress, scanty soft stools. For persons unable to tolerate rhubarb.

Cardamon and Fennel Formula with Major Rhubarb Combination or Coptis and Rhubarb Combination

Psychoneurosis, chills, stomach pain, chest distress, constipation

Minor Bupleurum Combination

Fatigability, loss of appetite, gastric distress, occasional nausea, constipation, stiff shoulders or tired back

Pinellia Combination

Stomach distress, nausea, vomiting or gas, a tendency towards diarrhea, occasional constipation with soft stools

Ginseng and Tang-kuei Formula

Chills with anemia, headache, stiff shoulders, lower back pain, and constipation

Minor Cinnamon and Paeonia Combination

Debilitated elderly people or babies with abdominal pain and constipation who suffer from abdominal pain after taking rhubarb

Major Zanthoxylum Combination

Abdominal chills and distress or constipation from hyperperistalsis

Rehmannia Eight Formula

Lower back pain or cold waist, urinary abnormalities, constipation

Vitality Combination

Severely cold feet and waist, diarrhea or successive soft stools, occasional constipation

Apricot and Linum Formula

Constipation with a ruddy complexion; fever; dry mouth and lips; fetid breath and a bitter taste in the mouth; a smooth, solid pulse; yellow fur on tongue with or without dryness

Astragalus Combination

Normal stools but difficult excretion; shortness of breath; a weak, soft pulse; light-colored tongue

Linum and Rhubarb Formula

Pale complexion and lips, constipation, vertigo, palpitations, thin tongue fur, a soft and small pulse

Pinellia and Sulphur Formula

Abdominal pain; difficult bowel movements; copious, transparent urine; fondness for heat; light tongue with white fur; a sinking, late pulse

XIV. Mental Instability and Insomnia

Bupleurum and Dragon Bone Combination

Severe psychoneurosis, excitability, sensation of periumbilical palpitation, constipation, insomnia

Persica and Rhubarb Combination

Headache, flushing, mental instability, cold feet and waist, lower back pain, constipation

Major Bupleurum Combination

Severe constipation, heart distress, mental instability, loss of vigor, a tendency to tire easily

Coptis and Rhubarb Combination

Flushing with severe constipation, gastric distress, mental instability, and insomnia

Cinnamon and Hoelen Formula

Flushing with headache, lower back pain, pain in the lower abdomen when palpated, dysmenorrhea, cold feet and waist, and psychoneurosis

Coptis and Scute Formula

Flushing with mental instability, a tendency to hemorrhage, and scanty stools

Minor Bupleurum Combination

Loss of appetite, malaise, anxiety, hot temper

Pinellia and Magnolia Combination

Psychoneurosis, unpleasant feeling in the pharynx or chest, mental instability, insomnia, nausea, vomiting, anorexia, fatigue, "hysteric ball" or the "running pig" syndrome, symptoms of Minor Bupleurum Combination

Cinnamon and Dragon Bone Combination

Tension in the lower abdomen, sensation of palpitation, sweating, psychoneurosis or fatigue

Ginseng and Gypsum Combination

Severe thirst, fever, an occasional hot feeling with psychoneurosis

Bupleurum, Cinnamon, and Ginger Combination

Poor health, malaise, weakness with night sweats, palpitation, dry lips, and fatigue

Cyperus and Perilla Formula

Severe psychoneurosis, headache, insomnia. For the elderly with delicate health.

Ma-huang and Magnolia Combination

Psychoneurotically-induced poor health, difficult breathing or cough, stridor with mental instability and insomnia

Tang-kuei and Gelatin Combination

Excessive hemorrhage or delayed and irregular menses, mental instability

Licorice and Jujube Combination

Alternate crying, laughing, and yawning

Hoelen, Licorice, and Jujube Combination
Severe "running pig" syndrome, palpitations beneath the umbilicus, severe abdominal pain

Pueraria and Ginger Combination
Paroxysmal abdominal pain, hysteric ball, absent-mindedness

XV. Edema

Atractylodes Combination
Acute and severe edema, thirst, decreased urinary volume, difficult breathing, a tendency to sweat

Minor Blue Dragon Combination
Watery sputum following coughing and subacute symptoms of Atractylodes Combination

Hoelen Five Herb Formula
Thirst, pronounced decrease in urinary volume, acute generalized edema

Ma-huang and Coix Combination
Chronic or subacute joint or muscular pain with occasional localized edema or a feverish feeling

Polyporus Combination
Scanty urination and a frequent feeling of urinary retention, thirst, occasional feverish feeling and edema in the lower body

Persica and Rhubarb Combination
Headache, stiff shoulders, cold lower body, lower back pain, abdominal pain when palpated, menstrual irregularity, constipation, edema of the feet or face, dark violet lips and nails

XVI. Fatigue

Ginseng Nutritive Combination
Chronic cough following debilitated health, heavy head, anorexia, and extreme fatigue

Ginseng and Astragalus Combination

Impaired digestion or--following illness--loss of appetite, extreme exhaustion, moderate fever, and anemia

Minor Cinnamon and Paeonia Combination

Poor health, susceptibility to colds, a tendency towards anemia, anorexia, abdominal pain, chills, abdominal distention, a predisposition toward diarrhea or constipation, weariness

Major Zanthoxylum Combination

Weak digestion, chills, abdominal distention, a tendency towards diarrhea or constipation, weariness

Cyperus and Perilla Formula

Psychoneurosis, headache, insomnia, fatigue. For elderly persons.

Rehmannia Eight Formula

Cold feet and waist with fever, decrease of urination, thirst, impaired vision, decreased vigor, lassitude

Pinellia and Magnolia Combination

Weakness from psychoneurosis, distressed feeling in the pharynx or dry cough, nausea, vomiting, fatigue

Ginseng and Tang-kuei Formula

Anemia, cold waist and feet, polyuria, heavy head, stiff shoulders, dizziness, lower back pain, a tendency to tire easily. If there is loss of appetite, one should add Minor Bupleurum Combination. For psychoneurosis add Pinellia and Magnolia Combination. For vertigo, Atractylodes and Hoelen Combination is prescribed additionally.

Minor Bupleurum Combination

Diseases of the endocrine glands; a tendency to tire; loss of appetite; stomach, thoracic, or abdominal distress; a predisposition to colds; chronic fever

Bupleurum and Dragon Bone Combination

Mental instability, insomnia, palpitation, psychoneurosis, malaise, constipation

Major Bupleurum Combination

Good health but severe constipation, abdominal and stomach distress, a tendency toward infirmity, and fatigue

XVII. Anorexia

Bupleurum and Cinnamon Combination

Severe pain in the chest, stomach, or abdomen or nausea or vomiting; heavy head with moderate fever; loss of appetite; night sweats

Capillaris Combination

Thoracic distress, thirst, head sweats, constipation with bloody stools, loss of appetite. With chronic or subacute symptoms, Hoelen Five Herb Formula is taken instead.

Major Bupleurum Combination

Good health, stomach distress with severe constipation, stiff shoulders, insomnia, fatigue, loss of appetite

Minor Bupleurum Combination

Diseases of the endocrine glands with a tendency to tire easily, chest or abdominal distress, moderate fever, nausea, vomiting, and loss of appetite

Bupleurum, Cinnamon, and Ginger Combination

Poor health with moderate fever, thirst, loss of appetite, night sweats, palpitation, asthma, and diarrhea or soft stools

Ginseng Nutritive Combination

Chronic cough or successive fever following debilitation, heavy head, anorexia, and night sweats

Magnolia and Ginger Formula

Gastric distress, loss of appetite, and impaired digestion, but a more comfortable feeling after diarrhea following meals

Pinellia Combination

Stomach distress, nausea, vomiting, loss of appetite, gas, soft stools

Cardamon and Fennel Formula

Psychoneurosis, gastric pain, cardiac distress, nausea, loss of appetite, chills. For constipation add rhubarb.

Pinellia and Magnolia Combination

Psychoneurosis and pharyngeal or thoracic distress, nausea, vomiting, dry cough, loss of appetite

Cyperus and Perilla Formula

Psychoneurosis. headache, stiff shoulders, insomnia, loss of appetite. Frail women or elderly men.

Hoelen Combination

Gastric distress with distention, nausea, anorexia, occasional dizziness or lower abdominal palpitation

Coptis and Scute Formula

A tendency to flush, stiff neck or shoulders, distressed stomach, loss of appetite, scanty stools

Minor Cinnamon and Paeonia Combination

Feeble health, a tendency toward anemia, susceptibility to fatigue, abdominal distention with pain, palpitation, loss of appetite

Ginseng and Astragalus Combination

Poor digestion, debilitation following sickness, loss of appetite, night sweats, moderate fever

Vitality Combination

Severely cold feet and waist, decreased urinary volume, heavy head, loss of appetite, vertigo, palpitation

Chapter Twelve

Important Chinese Herbal Prescriptions

Most of the basic formulas used in Chinese herbal medicine come from Chang Chung-ching's classics: *Treatise on Febrile Diseases* and *Summaries of Household Remedies.* Over the two thousand years of use, however, doctors and patients have altered and amended formulas and made up new ones.

Areca Seed Combination
(Chiu-pin-wu-fu-tang)

九檳吳茯湯

Objectives: beriberi, fatigue, weak legs, gasping, edema, swollen feeling under the heart, tendon pain, cardiac neurosis—difficult breathing, palpitation, insomnia, heart pain, nervousness, cold arms and legs, cold sweat, headache, diarrhea, and general body pain

Composition:

3.0g cinnamon twigs

3.0g Mandarin orange peel

4.0g betel seeds (areca)

3.0g ginger rhizome

3.0g magnolia bark

3.0g China root (hoelen)

Atractylodes Combination
(Yueh-pi-chia-chu-tang)

越婢加朮湯

Objectives: dry throat, edema or severe bullae, and occasional excessive secretion

Indications: nephritis, nephrosis, beriberi, arthritis, rheumatism, dermatitis, eczema, dacryocystitis, colitis, ocular eczema, keratitis, glaucoma, and nocturia

Composition:

6.0g ma-huang

8.0g gypsum

3.0g ginger rhizome

3.0g jujube fruit

2.0g licorice root

4.0g *paichu* (white atractylodes rhizome)

Atractylodes and Hoelen Combination
(Ling-kuei-chu-kan-tang)

苓桂朮甘湯

Objectives: dizziness, severe palpitation, flushing, headache, facial redness, anemia, increased urinary frequency but decreased volume, and dry lips.

Indications: tuberculosis, irregular pulse, cardiac neurosis, valvular disease, hypertension, hypotension, weakness, hysteria, conjunctivitis, ocular eczema or bleeding, corneal inflammation, dacryocystitis, cataract, rhinitis, suppuration, and Ménière's syndrome

Composition:

6.0g China root (hoelen)

4.0g cinnamon twigs

2.0g licorice root

3.0g *paichu* (white atractylodes rhizome)

Bupleurum and Cinnamon Combination
(Chai-hu-kuei-chih-tang)

柴胡桂枝湯

Objectives: sweating, slight fever, chills, distressed heart, headache, joint and occasional stomach pain, nausea, and severe abdominal pain with loss of appetite

Indications: cold pleurisy, gastric spasm or ulcer, cholelithiasis, cholecystitis, appendicitis, nephritis, nephrosis, pyelonephritis, petechiae, and intercostal neuralgia

Composition:

5.0g hare's ear root (bupleurum)

2.0g skullcap root (scute)

2.5g peony root

1.0g ginger rhizome

4.0g pinellia rhizome

2.0g ginseng root

2.5g cinnamon twigs

2.0g jujube fruit

1.5g licorice root

Bupleurum, Cinnamon, and Ginger Combination
(Chai-hu-kuei-chih-kan-chiang-tang)

柴胡桂枝乾薑湯

Objectives: delicate health, moderate fever, head and night sweats, distressed chest, malaise, loss of appetite, periumbilical spasms, a tendency towards weakness, insomnia, soft stools, decreased urine, dry mouth, and dry cough

Indications: cold, tuberculosis, pleurisy, pulse irregularities, cardiac disorders, endocarditis, valvular disease, cardiac asthma, hepatitis, cholecystitis, pancreatitis, peritonitis, weakness, nephritis, nephrosis, anemia, goiter, insomnia, hysteria, menopausal problems, and allergies

Composition:

6.0g hare's ear root (bupleurum)

3.0g cinnamon twigs

2.0g ginger rhizome

3.0g snake gourd root (trichosanthes)

3.0g skullcap root (scute)

3.0g oyster shell

2.0g licorice root

Bupleurum and Dragon Bone Combination
(Chai-hu-chia-lung-ku-mu-li-tang)

柴胡加龍骨牡蠣湯

Objectives: mental instability with a tendency to be frightened, cardiac hyperfunction, chest distress, vertigo, flushing, insomnia, occasional periumbilical palpitation, heart distress with constipation, and decreased urine

Indications: cardiac distress, valvular disease, cardiac asthma, angina pectoris, arteriosclerosis, hypertension, nephritis, nephrosis, kidney atrophy, impotence, sexual neurasthenia, goiter, insomnia, noctiphobia, menopausal disorders, and glaucoma

Composition:

5.0g hare's ear root (bupleurum)

4.0g pinellia rhizome

2.5g skullcap root (scute)

2.5g ginger rhizome

2.5g jujube fruit

2.5g ginseng root

3.0g cinnamon twigs

2.5g oyster shell

3.0g China root (hoelen)

1.0g rhubarb rhizome

2.5 dragon bone

Bupleurum and Schizonepeta Formula
(Shih-wei-pai-tu-san)

十味敗毒散

Objectives: chronic symptoms with slight secretion

Indications: furuncles, anthrax, lymphadenitis, anal ulcers, eczema, hives, infected suppurative crusts, warts, facial boils, mastitis, styes, blepharitis, otitis externa or media, and rhinitis

Composition:

3.0g hare's ear root (bupleurum)	2.0g angelica root (*tang-kuei*)
3.0g balloon flower root (platycodon)	1.0g *chinchieh* herb (schizonepeta)
1.0g ginger rhizome	1.0g licorice root
3.0g China root (hoelen)	3.0g Szechuan lovage rhizome (cnidium)
2.0g siler root	1.0g Pseudocerasi bark (cherry bark)

Bupleurum and Scute Combination
(Chai-hsien-tang)

柴陷湯

Objective: chest or back pain or chest fluid, distressed chest or stomach, and occasional cough ·

Indications: bronchial dilation, bronchitis. pleurisy, and intercostal neuralgia

Composition:

5.0g hare's ear root (bupleurum)	1.5g licorice root
3.0g skullcap root (scute)	5.0g pinellia rhizome
3.0g ginger rhizome	3.0g snake gourd fruit and seeds (trichosanthes)
3.0g jujube fruit	
2.0g ginseng root	1.5g goldenthread rhizome (coptis)

Capillaris Combination
(Yin-chen-hao-tang)

茵陳蒿湯

Objectives: dry throat, chest distress with constipation—suitable for patients with jaundice

Indications: hepatitis, nephritis, nephrosis, hives, and stomatitis

Composition:

1.0g capillary artemisia herb	1.0g rhubarb rhizome
2.0g gardenia fruit	

Cardamon and Fennel Formula
(An-chung-san)

安中散

Objectives: chills and psychoneurosis with stomach pain or heart distress

Indications: gastritis, prolapsed and weak stomach, and gastric and duodenal ulcers

Composition:

4.0g cinnamon twigs	0.5g lesser galangal rhizome
3.0g corydalis rhizome	0.5 licorice root
3.0g oyster shell	1.0g cardamon seeds
1.5g fennel fruit	

Cimicifuga Combination
(I-tzu-tang)

乙字湯

Objectives: constipation with minor bleeding, severe local pain

Indications: hemorrhoids, prolapsed rectum, and vaginal itching

Composition:

1.0g rhubarb rhizome	2.0g licorice root
6.0g Chinese angelica root (*tang-kuei*)	5.0g hare's ear root (bupleurum)
3.0g skullcap root (scute)	1.5g bugbane rhizome (cimicifuga)

Cinnamon Combination
(Kuei-chih-tang)

桂枝湯

Objectives: chills, fever, headache, weak pulse, and sweating. It is good for those of delicate health.

Indications: colds, neuralgia, headache, rheumatism, abdominal pain, neurasthenia, impotence, and emissions

Composition:

4.0g cinnamon twigs	4.0g ginger rhizome
4.0g jujube fruit	2.0g licorice root
4.0g peony root	

Cinnamon, Atractylodes, and Aconite Combination
(Kuei-chih-chia-chu-fu-tang)

桂枝加尤附湯

Objectives: chilled and numb feeling with pain or difficulty moving

Indications: neuralgia, rheumatism, stiff shoulders in persons over fifty, and paralysis on one side

Composition:

4.0g cinnamon twigs	2.0g licorice root
4.0g peony root	4.0g paichu (white atractylodes rhizome)
4.0g ginger rhizome	1.0g mugwort root (aconite)
4.0g jujube fruit	

Cinnamon, Hoelen, and Atractylodes Combination
(Kuei-chih-chia-ling-chu-tang)

桂枝加苓尤湯

Objectives: same as for Cinnamon Combination along with palpitation and difficult urination

Indications: heart failure, ear and digestive disorders, beriberi, ocular neuralgia, lower back pain, rheumatism, and arthritis

Composition:

4.0g cinnamon twigs	5.0g paichu (white atractylodes rhizome)
3.0g peony root	3.0g jujube fruit
3.0g ginger rhizome	1.5g licorice root
5.0g China root (hoelen)	

Cinnamon and Dragon Bone Combination
(Kuei-chih-chia-lung-ku-mu-li-tang)

桂枝加龍骨牡蠣湯

Objectives: psychoneurosis with headache, flushing, tinnitus, tendency to fatigue, spasms at the umbilicus, and polyuria

Indications: sexual weakness, nocturia, night fears, falling hair, and penile atrophy

Composition:

4.0g cinnamon twigs	2.0g licorice root
4.0g peony root	3.0g dragon bone
4.0g ginger rhizome	3.0g oyster shell
4.0g jujube fruit	

Cinnamon and Hoelen Formula
(Kuei-chih-fu-ling-wan)

桂枝茯苓丸

Objectives: flushing, headache, stiff shoulders, dizziness with chills, and pain in the
lower abdomen

Indications: difficult menstruation, endometritis, swelling of uterine muscles, oophoritis, salpingitis, menopausal disorders, sterility, orchitis, appendicitis, hepatitis,
arthritis, sciatic neuralgia, chilblains, hemorrhoids, eczema, hives, facial vesicles,
maculae, styes, ocular eczema, and iritis

Composition:

4.0g cinnamon twigs	4.0g tree peony bark
4.0g peony root	4.0g peach seeds (persica)
4.0g China root (hoelen)	

Cinnamon and Peony Combination
(Kuei-chih-chia-shao-yao-tang)

桂枝加芍藥湯

Objectives: abdominal distress with frequent pain—usually periumbilical or in lower
abdomen; diarrhea with muddy and mucous stools while suffering from a cold;
abdominal pain; intestinal catarrh; peritonitis with nodules; acute or chronic
appendicitis—unsuitable for peritonitis with fluid and exudate

Indications: delicate health, diarrhea from weakness, abdominal distention and pain

Composition:

4.0g cinnamon twigs	2.0g licorice root
6.0g peony root	4.0g jujube fruit
4.0g ginger rhizome	

Cnidium and Rhubarb Formula
(Chiung-huang-san)

芎黄散

Objectives: moderate purgative for habitual constipation in the elderly or persons
with delicate health

Indications: constipation, headache, and heavy head

Composition:

1.1g Chinese lovage rhizome (cnidium)   1.0g rhubarb rhizome

Coix Combination
(I-yi-jen-tang)

薏苡仁湯

Objectives: general pain in the muscles and joints, numbness, pain in the feet and hands, and stiffness occasionally associated with swelling or fever. Also for stiff shoulders caused by extravasated blood or cold.

Indications: neuralgia, rheumatism, and arthritis

Composition:

8.0g Job's tears seeds (coix)

4.0g Chinese angelica root (*tang-kuei*)

3.0g cinnamon twigs

2.0g licorice

4.0g ma-huang herb

4.0g *paichu* (white atractylodes rhizome)

3.0g peony root

Coptis and Rhubarb Combination
(San-huang-hsieh-hsin-tang)

三黃瀉心湯

Objectives: flushing, mental instability, stomach distress with severe constipation, and an occasional tendency towards hyperemia or hemorrhaging

Indications: hemoptysis, hemorrhoidal bleeding, chronic constipation, hypertension, arteriosclerosis, excessive or vicarious menstruation, conjunctivitis, cataract, and eye hemorrhage

Composition:

1.0g goldenthread rhizome (coptis)

1.0g skullcap root (scute)

1.0g rhubarb rhizome

Coptis and Scute Combination
(Huang-lien-chieh-tu-tang)

黃連解毒湯

Objectives: flushing, distressed stomach or soft stools with constipation, and ocular hyperemia

Indications: tuberculosis, stomatitis, gastritis, hemoptysis, intestinal, uterine or hemorrhoidal bleeding, hepatitis, hypertension, weakness, insomnia, and bleeding eyelids

Composition:

3.0g goldenthread root (coptis)

2.0g skullcap root (scute)

2.0g phellodendron bark

1.0g gardenia fruit

Cyperus and Perilla Formula
(Hsiang-su-san)

香蘇散

Objectives: psychoneurosis, headache, melancholia, and loss of appetite
Indications: cold, headache, migraine, hives, hysteria, menopausal disorders, and difficult menstruation
Composition:

4.0g nutgrass rhizome (cyperus)	3.0g ginger rhizome
1.0g perilla leaf	1.0g licorice root
2.5g citrus peel	

Dragon Bone and Oyster Shell Combination
(Lung-ku-mu-li-tang)

龍骨牡蠣湯

Objectives: a sedative for palpitation and an astringent for night sweats
Indications: hypersecretion of gastric acid, neuralgia, chronic gastritis, and difficult urination
Composition:

1.0g dragon bone	1.0g oyster shell
0.1g gum arabic	

Eriocheir and Viper Formulas
(Po-chou-san)

伯州散

Objectives: subacute or chronic dermatosis with suppuration
Indications: bone ulcers, nodules, crusts, anal ulcers, hemorrhoids, dermatosis with suppuration, mastitis, dacryocystitis, otitis media, and gum abscess
Composition:

1.0g eriocheir	1.0g deer horn
1.0g viper	

Ginseng and Astragalus Combination
(Pu-chung-i-chi-tang)

補中益氣湯

Objectives: decreased stomach and intestinal function; fatigue, severe loss of appetite;

and occasional headache, chills, night sweats, and slow bleeding

Indications: tuberculosis; pleurisy; weak digestion; prolapsed stomach, rectum, or uterus; peritonitis; hypotension; involuntary emission; impotence; anemia; hysteria; insomnia; osseous ulcers; endometritis; and increased sweating

Composition:

4.0g ginseng root

3.0g Chinese angelica

1.5g licorice root

4.0g *paichu* (white atractylodes rhizome)

2.0g Mandarin orange peel

1.0g hare's ear root (bupleurum)

0.5g bugbane rhizome (cimicifuga)

4.0g Chinese milk vetch root (astragalus)

0.5g ginger rhizome

Ginseng and Ginger Combination
(Jen-sheng-tang)

人參湯

Objectives: weak digestion, pale face, wet tongue, polyuria with low specific gravity, cold arms and legs, oversecretion of saliva, tendency towards diarrhea, occasional vomiting, dizziness, headache, gastric pain, irregular pulse, and abdominal distention

Indications: acute or chronic gastritis, weak digestion, stomach dilation, nausea, pale face from renal atrophy, edema, polyuria, tendency towards diarrhea, intoxication in children

Composition:

3.0g ginseng root

3.0g *paichu* rhizome (white atractylodes)

2.0-3.0g ginger rhizome

3.0g licorice root

Ginseng and Gypsum Combination
(Pai-hu-chia-jen-sheng-tang)

白虎加人參湯

Objectives: severe thirst with a constant desire to drink or a strong feverish sensation

Indications: diabetes mellitus, pneumonia, measles, sunstroke, and cold

Composition:

5.0g anemarrhena rhizome

15.0g gypsum

10.0g rice

2.0g licorice root

3.0g ginseng root

Ginseng Nutritive Combination
(Jen-sheng-yang-yung-tang)

人參養榮湯

Objectives: slender physique with chronic fever, chills, chronic cough, fatigue, loss of appetite, mental instability, night sweats, and tendency towards constipation

Indications: tuberculosis, pleurisy, penile atrophy after sickness, postpartum weakness, and constipation

Composition:

3.0g ginseng root	4.0g Chinese foxglove root
2.5g Chinese milk vetch root (astragalus)	and rhizome (rehmannia)
	4.0g peony root
4.0g white *paichu* rhizome (atractylodes)	2.5g citrus peel
	2.0g Chinese milkwort root (polygala)
4.0g China root (hoelen)	1.5g schizandra fruit
4.0g Chinese angelica root (*tang-kuei*)	1.5g licorice root
2.5g cinnamon twigs	

Ginseng and Tang-kuei Formula
(Jen-sheng-tang-shao-san)

人參當芍散

Objectives: cold arms and legs, psychoneurosis, dry skin, tired eyes, headache, dizziness, tinnitus, menopausal complaints, weakness, stiff shoulders, and neurasthenia

Indications: chronic nephritis, kidney disease during pregnancy, and lower back pain

Composition:

3.0g Chinese angelica root (*tang-kuei*)	3.0g *paichu* rhizome (white atractylodes rhizome)
2.5g Chinese lovage rhizome (cnidium)	
3.0g peony root	3.0g China root (hoelen)
3.0g water plantain rhizome (alisma)	3.0g ginseng root
1.5g cinnamon twigs	1.0g licorice root

Hoelen Combination
(Fu-ling-yin)

茯苓飲

Objectives: distressed stomach with swollen feeling, hypersecretion of gastric fluid, nausea, loss of appetite, and decreased urine

Indications: prolapsed stomach, weak digestion, gastric disorders, and stomach dilation

Composition:

5.0g China root (hoelen)	3.0g ginger rhizome
4.0g *paichu* rhizome (white atractylodes rhizome)	1.5g immature citrus peel
	3.0g Mandarin orange peel
3.0g ginseng root	

Hoelen Five Herb Formula
(Wu-ling-san)

五苓散

Objectives: excessive dry throat, decreased urinary volume, heavy head, head sweats, nausea, vomiting—occasionally associated with swelling

Indications: watery dysentery, acute gastroenteric catarrh, vomiting, drunkenness, sunstroke, hepatitis, cirrhosis of the liver, jaundice, cholelithiasis, cholecystitis, peritonitis, valvular diseases, nephritis, nephrosis, pyelonephritis, cystitis, urethritis, diabetes mellitus, trigeminal neuralgia, dacryocystitis, and night blindness

Composition:

3.0g cinnamon twigs	6.5g China root (hoelen)
4.5g *paichu* (white atractylodes rhizome)	6.0g water plantain rhizome (alisma)
4.5g grifola (polyporus)	

Hoelen and Ginger Combination
(Ling-chiang-chu-kan-tang)

苓薑朮甘湯

Objectives: cold waist and feet, pain, fatigue, polyuria, and cold sweat or watery secretions

Indications: lower back pain, cold waist and feet, sciatic neuralgia, leukorrhea, urinary retention, nocturia in children, eczema, and ulcers

Composition:

6.0g China root (hoelen)	3.0g *paichu* (white atractylodes rhizome)
3.0g ginger rhizome	2.0g licorice root

Lithospermum Ointment
(Tzu-yun-kao)
紫雲膏

Objectives: to promote granulation of tissue and to prevent dermal erosion
Indications: burns, chilblain, anal ulcers, hemorrhoids, facial vesicles, infected crusts, and athlete's foot
Composition:

100.0g Chinese angelica root (*tang-kuei*)	1000.0g flax oil
100.0g Asiatic groomwell root	25.0g lard
(lithospermum)	380.0g beeswax

Magnolia and Ginger Formula
(Ping-wei-san)
平胃散

Objectives: stomach pain with indigestion, abdominal discomfort, diarrhea, loss of appetite, and gas after meals; relief follows diarrhea
Indications: stomatitis, gastritis, weak digestion, gastric dilation, and diarrhea
Composition:

3.0g magnolia bark	1.0g ginger rhizome
4.0g *tsangchu* (atractylodes rhizome)	1.0g licorice root
3.0g Mandarin orange peel	2.0g jujube fruit

Ma-huang Combination
(Ma-huang-tang)
麻黃湯

Objectives: severe fever or chills with pain, rheumatoid discomfort, stuffy nose in infants, and acute dermal suppuration
Indications: influenza, bronchitis, bronchial asthma, pneumonia, rhinitis, acute arthritis, muscular rheumatism, stuffy nose, and acute dermatosis in infancy with suppuration
Composition:

5.0g ma-huang herb	1.5g licorice root
4.0g cinnamon twigs	5.0g apricot seeds

Ma-huang and Apricot Seed Combination
(Ma-hsing-kan-shih-tang)

麻杏甘石湯

Objectives: severe cough with dry throat, head sweating, and stridor
Indications: bronchitis, whooping cough, bronchial and childhood asthma, and pneumonia
Composition:

4.0g ma-huang herb	10.0g gypsum
2.0g licorice root	4.0g apricot seeds

Ma-huang and Asarum Combination
(Ma-huang-hsi-hsin-fu-tzu-tang)

麻黃細辛附子湯

Objectives: moderate fever, fatigue, headache, chills, and body pain
Indications: delicate health, colds in the elderly, bronchitis, acute fever, asthma, suppuration, and cough from poor health
Composition:

4.0g ma-huang herb (ephedra)	1.0g wolfsbane root (aconite)
3.0g wild ginger herb (asarum)	

Ma-huang and Coix Combination
(Ma-hsing-i-kan-tang)

麻杏薏甘湯

Objectives: acute or chronic arthritis and muscular pain
Indications: joint and muscular rheumatism, warts, athlete's foot, chronic nephritis, and nephritis in pregnancy
Composition:

4.0g ma-huang herb	10.0g Job's tears seeds (coix)
3.0g apricot seeds	2.0g licorice root

Ma-huang and Magnolia Combination
(Shen-mi-tang)

神秘湯

Objectives: chronic cough with small volume of sputum
Indications: bronchial asthma

Composition:

5.0g ma-huang herb	2.5g citrus peel
4.0g apricot seeds	3.0g magnolia bark
2.0g licorice root	2.0g bupleurum root
1.5g perilla leaves	

Major Bupleurum Combination
(Ta-chai-hu-tang)　　大柴胡湯

Objectives: heart distress, pain and pressure in the chest or around the abdomen, severe constipation, occasional tinnitus aurium, stiff shoulders, and loss of appetite

Indications: bronchial asthma, gastritis, gastric or duodenal ulcer, chronic dysentery, habitual constipation, hepatitis, cholelithiasis, cholecystitis, hypertension, arteriosclerosis, insomnia, involuntary emission, impotence, sexual neurasthenia, obesity, diabetes mellitus, intercostal neuralgia, furunculosis, anthrax, bleeding hemorrhoids, rectocele, eczema, hives, facial vesicles, keratitis, iritis, tinnitus aurium, otitis media, suppuration, tonsillitis, and alveolar pyorrhea

Composition:

6.0g hare's ear root (bupleurum)	2.0g immature citrus peel
3.0g skullcap root (scute)	1.0-2.0g rhubarb rhizome
4.0g pinellia rhizome	3.0g jujube fruit
3.0g peony root	4.0g ginger rhizome

Minor Blue Dragon Combination
(Hsiao-ching-lung-tang)　　小青龍湯

Objectives: decreased urinary volume after acute fever, chest distress, sensation of fluid in the stomach, coughing of watery sputum with stridor or rhinitis with copious nasal drainage, and opthalmological disorders with tearing

Indications: bronchitis, rhinitis, bronchial asthma, whooping cough, bronchial enlargement, pleurisy, nephritis, nephrosis, arthritis, conjunctivitis, ocular eczema, keratitis, and dacryocystitis

Composition:

3.0g ma-huang herb	3.0g wild ginger root (asarum)

3.0g peony root

3.0g ginger rhizome

3.0g licorice root

3.0g schizandra fruit

3.0g cinnamon twigs

6.0g pinellia rhizome

Minor Bupleurum Combination
(Hsiao-chai-hu-tang)

小柴胡湯

Objectives: distressed chest or abdomen, slight fever with alternating chills, loss of appetite with bitter taste, occasional white tongue coating, nausea, vomiting, and cough

Indications: cold, bronchitis, whooping cough, bronchial and childhood asthma, pneumonia, tuberculosis, pleurisy, gastritis, stomach and duodenal ulcers, hepatitis, cirrhosis of the liver, cholelithiasis, cholecystitis, pancreatitis, peritonitis, nephritis, nephrosis, pyelonephritis, kidney and gall stones, anemia, tonsillitis, otitis media, measles, childbirth fever, mastitis, ocular eczema, keratitis, iritis, rhinitis, and suppuration

Composition:

7.0g hare's ear root (bupleurum)

3.0g skullcap root (scute)

5.0g pinellia rhizome

4.0g ginger rhizome

3.0g jujube fruit

2.0g licorice root

3.0g ginseng root

Minor Cinnamon and Peony Combination
(Hsiao-chien-chung-tang)

小建中湯

Objectives: poor health with a tendency toward fatigue, flushing, abdominal pain or palpitation, chills with warm arms and legs, frequent urination

Indications: gastroptosis, indigestion, reduction of acid, childhood dysentery, peritonitis, childhood constipation, rickets, noctiphobia, nocturia, bone ulcers, prolapsed rectum, ocular eczema, keratitis, iritis, and tonsillitis

Composition:

4.0g cinnamon twigs

6.0g peony root

2.0g licorice root

4.0g ginger rhizome

4.0g jujube fruit

20.0g maltose

Ophiopogon Combination
(Mai-men-tung-tang)

麥門冬湯

Objectives: cough with flushing up and usually a small volume of sticky sputum, or flushing up with dryness and odd sensation in the throat

Indications: bronchitis, whooping cough, bronchial or childhood asthma, laryngitis, pneumonia, tuberculosis, and diabetes mellitus

Composition:

5.0g pinellia rhizome	10.0g ophiopogon root
2.0g ginseng root	2.0g licorice root
3.0g jujube fruit	5.0g rice

Peony and Licorice Combination
(Shao-yao-kan-tsao-tang)

芍藥甘草湯

Objectives: muscular pain and tension, pain in the feet, and muscular rheumatism; bronchial asthma; pain in the abdomen; and cholelithiasis

Indications: rheumatoid pain, sciatic neuralgia, and lower back pain

Composition:

4.0-8.0g peony root	4.0-8.0g licorice

Persica and Rhubarb Combination
(Tao-ho-cheng-chi-tang)

桃核承氣湯

Objectives: violet or dark pink lips or gums, and tendency toward headaches or flushing

Indications: habitual constipation, hypertension, arteriosclerosis, nephritis, nephrosis, kidney atrophy, cystitis, enlarged prostate, hypertrophy, sciatic neuralgia, chilblains, hemorrhoids, menstrual disorders, endometritis, swelling of uterine muscles, oophoritis, salpingitis, menopausal disorders, eczema, hives, facial vesicles, tinea, ocular eczema, iritis, glaucoma, ocular bleeding, periodentitis, and alveodental suppuration

Composition:

5.0g peach seeds (persica)	1.5g licorice root
4.0g cinnamon twigs	2.0g nitrous sulfate
3.0g rhubarb rhizome	

151

Pinellia Combination
(Pan-hsia-hsieh-hsin-tang)

半夏瀉心湯

Objectives: distressed stomach, nausea, and vomiting

Indications: prolapsed stomach, stomatitis, gastritis, weak digestion, diarrhea, enteritis, nausea, gastric and duodenal ulcers

Composition:

1.0g goldenthread rhizome (coptis)	3.0g jujube fruit
3.0g skullcap root (scute)	3.0g licorice root
6.0g pinellia rhizome	3.0g ginger roots
3.0g ginseng root	

Pinellia and Ginseng Six Combination
(Pan-hsieh-liu-chun-tzu-tang)

半瀉六君子湯

Objectives: distended or tense stomach, pain, nausea, distressed heart, gas, diarrhea, anemia, loss of appetite, vomiting, fatigue, painful hunger, and gastric spasms or dilation

Indications: gastric or intestinal catarrh, hypersecretion of gastric acid, prolapsed stomach, stomach and duodenal ulcers, and gastric weakness

Composition:

4.0g pinellia rhizome	3.0g licorice root
4.0g ginseng root	9.0g China root (hoelen)
3.0g skullcap root (scute)	3.0g *paichu* (white atractylodes rhizome)
3.0g goldenthread rhizome (coptis)	3.0g Mandarin orange peel
1.0g ginger rhizome	4.0g oyster shell

Pinellia and Magnolia Combination
(Pan-hsia-hou-pu-tang)

半夏厚朴湯

Objectives: mental instability, distressed throat and chest, stomach distention, weak digestion, occasional nausea, and vomiting

Indications: bronchitis, tonsillitis, pharyngitis, whooping cough, bronchial asthma, tuberculosis, esophageal stricture, gastric neurosis, poor digestion, prolapsed stomach, irregular pulse, cardiac nerve disorders, cardiac asthma, hypotension, neurasthenia, phobias, insomnia, nausea, menopausal disorders, uterine bleeding, and absence of menses

Composition:

6.0g pinellia rhizome

5.0g China root (hoelen)

3.0g magnolia bark

2.0g perilla leaves

4.0g ginger rhizome

Platycodon and Chih-shih Formula
(Pai-nung-san)

排膿散

Indications: tumors with suppuration and pain, muscle spasms, nodules, crusts, and lymphadenitis. Note: Unsuitable for chronic tumors and cold sores.

Composition:

5.0g immature citrus fruit (*chih-shih*)   2.0g balloon flower root (platycodon)

5.0g peony root

Platycodon and Gypsum Combination
(Chieh-keng-shih-kao-tang)

桔梗石膏湯

Objectives: thirst and chronic expectoration

Indications: expectoration

Composition:

1.1g balloon flower root (platycodon)   1.0g gypsum

Polyporus Combination
(Chu-ling-tang)

豬苓湯

Objectives: dry throat, painful urination, dysuria, and hematuria

Indications: pyelonephritis, kidney or gall stones, cystitis, urethritis, and gonorrhea

Composition:

3.0g water plantain rhizome (alisma)

3.0g China root (hoelen)

3.0g talc

3.0g grifola (polyporus)

3.0g gelatin

Pueraria Combination
(Ko-ken-tang)

葛根湯

Objectives: headache; fever; chills without sweating; pain in the neck, shoulders, and back; chronic dental pain; stuffy nose; suppuration; stiff shoulders; and neuralgia

Indications: cold, otitis media, rhinitis, suppuration, trachoma, tonsillitis, styes, conjunctivitis, ocular eczema, iritis, dacryocystitis, cataract, eczema, hives, mastitis, alveodental suppuration, measles, trigeminal neuralgia, muscular rheumatism, enteritis, and hemicrania

Composition:

8.0g common kudzu root (pueraria)	3.0g cinnamon twigs
4.0g ma-huang herb	3.0g peony root
1.0g ginger rhizome	2.0g licorice root
4.0g jujube fruit	

Pueraria Nasal Combination
(Ching-pi-tan₅)

清鼻湯

Indications: stuffy nose, headache, chronic nasal suppuration, supraorbital neuralgia, melancholia, rhinitis, and postoperative nasal diseases

Composition:

Pueraria Combination	gypsum
Cnidium and Rhubarb Formula	Job's tears seeds (coix)
balloon flower root	magnolia flowers
(platycodon)	

Rehmannia Eight Formula
(Pa-wei-ti-huang-wan)

八味地黃丸

Objectives: a tendency towards fatigue; cold, or sometimes hot, arms and legs; occasional lower back pain; dry throat; frequent urination with decreased volume and sensation of retention; and occasional polyuria at night

Indications: hypertension, arteriosclerosis, nephritis, nephrosis, kidney atrophy, pyelitis, kidney and gall stones, urethritis, enlargement of the prostate, involuntary emissions, impotence, genital neuralgia, beriberi after childbirth, menopausal disorders, eczema, hives, weak eyesight, cataract, glaucoma, and pyorrhea

Composition:

- 4.0g yam (dioscorea)
- 4.0g Asiatic cornelian cherry fruit (cornus)
- 3.0g water plantain rhizome (alisma)
- 3.0g China root (hoelen)
- 1.0g cinnamon twigs
- 8.0g Chinese foxglove roots and rhizome (rehmannia)
- 1.0g wolfsbane root (aconite)
- 3.0g tree peony bark

Rhubarb and Moutan Combination
(Ta-huang-mu-tan-pi-tang)

大黃牡丹皮湯

Objectives: distressed pain or constipation of the upper colon, hard stools, purplish or dark red skin, hyperemia, or tendency to bleed

Indications: appendicitis, chronic constipation, arteriosclerosis, kidney or gall stones, cystitis, urethritis, enlarged prostate, tendonitis, menstrual irregularity, endometritis, oopharitis, salpingitis, orchitis, menopausal problems, eczema, facial vesicles, ringworm, infected crusts, and iritis

Composition:

- 2.0g rhubarb rhizome
- 4.0g nitrous sulfate
- 4.0g tree peony bark (moutan)
- 6.0g wax gourd seeds
- 4.0g peach seeds

Rhubarb Five Formula
(Wu-huang-san)

五黃散

Objectives: flushing, dark red face, distressed heart, mental instability, occasional insomnia, dizziness, stiff shoulders, and a rough feeling in the mouth

Indications: hypertension, arteriosclerosis, tinnitus, stiff shoulders, stomach ulcer, gastritis, menopausal disorders, insomnia, nosebleed, uterine bleeding, headache from habitual constipation, hyperemia, dry lips, bitter tongue, and alcoholism

Composition:

- 4.5g goldenthread rhizome (coptis)
- 9.0g rhubarb rhizome
- 3.5g skullcap root (scute)
- 3.5g phellodendron bark
- 3.5g gardenia fruit

Siler and Platycodon Formula
(Fang-feng-tung-sheng-san)

防風通聖散

Objectives: obesity with constipation and decreased urine volume

Indications: stomach and duodenal ulcers, habitual constipation, irregular pulse, cardiac neurosis, angina pectoris, valvular disease, cardiac asthma, fatty heart, arteriosclerosis, hypertension, nephrosis, kidney and bladder stones, involuntary emission, impotence, sexual weakness, obesity, stiff shoulders in persons over fifty, arthritis, neuralgia, nodules, crusty skin, eczema, hives, rosacea, athlete's foot, loss of hair, corneal inflammation, iritis, cataract, otitis media, suppuration and gingival abscess

Composition:

1.2g Chinese angelica root (*tang-kuei*)
1.2g Chinese lovage rhizome (cnidium)
1.2g peony root
1.2g gardenia fruit
1.2g ginger rhizome
1.2g forsythia fruit
3.0g siler root
2.0g licorice root
1.2g *chinchieh* herb (schizonepeta))
1.5g nitrous sulfate

1.2g ma-huang herb (ephedra)
2.0g *paichu* (white atractylodes rhizome)
1.5g rhubarb rhizome
1.2g field mint herb
2.0g balloon flower root (platycodon)
2.0g skullcap root (scute)
2.0g gypsum
3.0g talc

Sophora and Schizonepeta Formula
(Ku-chin-san)

苦荊散

Indications: eczema

Composition:

1.0g sophora root

1.0g *chinchieh* herb (schizonepeta)

Stephania and Astragalus
(Fang-chi-huang-chi-tang)

防己黃耆湯

Objectives: edema; clear, pale skin; and a tendency toward swelling and sweating

Indications: obesity, arthritis, joint rheumatism, and sweating

Composition:

5.0g stephania root

5.0g Chinese milk vetch root
   (astragalus)

3.0g ginger rhizome

3.0g *paichu* (white atractylodes
   rhizome)

3.0g jujube fruit

1.5g licorice root

Stephania and Ginseng Combination
(Mu-fang-chi-tang)

木防己湯

Objectives: distressed heart, difficult breathing with asthmatic breath sounds, occasional edematous swelling with decreased urine, and thirst

Indications: endocarditis, valvular diseases, cardiac asthma, chronic nephritis, and nephrosis

Composition:

4.0g stephania root

3.0g ginseng

10.0g gypsum

3.0g cinnamon twigs

Tang-kuei and Arctium Formula
(Hsiao-feng-san)

消風散

Objectives: chronic dry or secreting dermatosis which aggravates during summer or warm weather

Indications: hives and eczema

Composition:

3.0g Chinese angelica root (*tang-kuei*)

3.0g Chinese foxglove root and
   rhizome (rehmannia)

3.0g gypsum

2.0g siler root

2.0g *tsangchu* rhizome (atractylodes)

1.0g *chinchieh* herb (schizonepeta)

2.0g birthwort

2.0g burdock (arctium)

1.5g anemarrhena rhizome

1.5g flax seeds

1.0g cicada

1.0g sophora root

Tang-kuei and Bupleurum Formula
(Hsiao-yao-san)

逍遙散

Objectives: tendency toward fatigue, headache, stiff shoulders, dizziness, chest distress, red face with hot sensation, turbid urine, urinary retention, bad temper, and mental instability

Indications: women with delicate health; psychoneurosis, neurasthenia, hysteria, insomnia, menstrual irregularity, tuberculosis, dermatosis, leukorrhea, chronic endometritis, and hypertensive palpitation

Composition:

3.0g Chinese angelica root (tang-kuei)	3.0g paichu (white atractylodes rhizome)
3.0g peony root	2.0g ginger rhizome
3.0g hare's ear root (bupleurum)	1.5g licorice root
3.0g China root (hoelen)	1.0g field mint

Tang-kuei, Evodia, and Ginger Combination
(Tang-kuei-szu-ni-chia-wu-chu-yu-sheng-chiang-tang)

當歸四逆加吳茱萸生薑湯

Objectives: severely cold arms and legs, tendency towards anemia, and occasional chills with lower back pain or lower abdominal pain

Indications: sciatic neuralgia, chilblains, and lower abdominal pain in women

Composition:

3.0g Chinese angelica root (tang-kuei)	2.0g asarum
3.0g cinnamon twigs	3.0g akebia
3.0g peony root	5.0g jujube fruit
2.0g licorice root	2.0g evodia fruit
4.0g ginger rhizome	

Tang-kuei Four Combination
(Szu-wu-tang)

四物湯

Objectives: one of the choicest drugs for gynecological problems; used for anemia and as a tranquilizer for psychosomatic complaints

Indications: menstrual irregularity, menopausal disorders, leukorrhea, pre- or post-partum illnesses

Composition:

4.0g Chinese angelica root (*tang-kuei*) 4.0g peony root

4.0g Chinese lovage rhizome (cnidium) 4.0g Chinese foxglove roots and rhizome (rehmannia)

Tang-kuei and Gelatin Combination
(*Chiung-kuei-chiao-ai-tang*)

芎歸膠艾湯

Objectives: chills and anemia from excessive bleeding

Indications: hemoptysis, metrorrhagia, intestinal or hemorrhoidal bleeding, hemorrhage during pregnancy, chronic bleeding after childbirth, excessive menstruation, and petechiae

Composition:

4.5g Chinese angelica root (*tang-kuei*) 6.0g rehmannia roots and rhizome

3.0g Chinese lovage rhizome (cnidium) 3.0g licorice root

4.5g peony root 3.0g mugwort leaves (artemisia)

3.0g gelatin

Tang-kuei and Paeonia Formula
(*Tang-kuei-shao-yao-san*)

當歸芍藥散

Objectives: anemia with chills, pallor, dark color around the eyes, headache, dizziness, stiff shoulders, palpitation, urinary frequency but small volume, thirst, and pain or chills in the lower abdomen

Indications: irregular pulse, cardiac neurosis, valvular disease, hypotension, hypertension, nephritis, nephrosis, anemia, goiter, chilblains, hemorrhoids, prolapsed rectum or uterus, habitual abortion, nephritis in pregnancy, periodic menstrual irregularity, retroverted uterus, endometritis, congenital abnormalities, sterility, menopausal problems, hysteria, facial vesicles, athlete's feet, ringworm, ocular eczema, iritis, dacrycystitis, and cataract

Composition:

3.0g Chinese angelica root (*tang-kuei*) 4.0g water plantain rhizome (alisma)

3.0g Chinese lovage rhizome (cnidium) 4.0g *paichu* (white atractylodes rhizome)

4.0g peony root (paeonia) 4.0g China root (hoelen)

Vitality Combination
(Chen-wu-tang)

眞武湯

Objectives: severely cold arms and legs, decreased urine, a tendency towards diarrhea, palpitation, and dizziness

Indications: chronic diarrhea, prolapsed stomach, peritonitis, appendicitis, hypertension, arteriosclerosis, and hypotension

Composition:

3.0g peony root

3.0g ginger rhizome

5.0g China root (hoelen)

3.0g *paichu* (white atractylodes rhizome)

1.0g wolfsbane root (aconite)

Chapter Thirteen

Commonly Used Herbs

Achyranthes

Botanical name: *Achyranthes bidentata, Cya-thula capitata* (Amaranthaceae)

Pharmaceutical name: Radix Achyranthis

Chinese Name: *niu-hsi* 牛膝

From *Shen Nung's Herbal* (superior drug)

Constituents: saponin

Properties and actions: neutral, bitter, and acrid to taste. Beneficial to the liver and kidneys; strengthens the muscles and bone structure; promotes menstrual regularity, diuresis, and pus drainage; and resolves bruises.

Indications: amenorrhea, gonorrhea, hematuria, swelling carbuncles, dystocia, stagnant blood, weakness of the liver and kidneys, pain in the waist and knees, and generalized weakness.

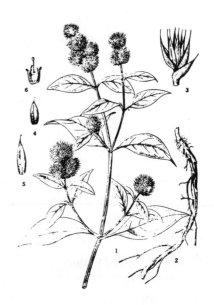

Cyathula capitata

161

Aconite
(Monkshood; Wolfsbane)

Botanical name: *Aconitum carmichaeli, A. chinense, A. coreahum, A. sinense, A. sanyonse, A. napellus* (Ranunculaceae)

Pharmaceutical name: Radix Aconiti, Radix Aconiti Carmichaeli Praeparata

Chinese name: *ch'uan-wu, tsao-wu, fu-tzu* 川烏，草烏；附子

Constituents: picroaconitine, aconine, aconitic acid, starch, fat, resin, benzoic acid

Properties and actions: slightly warm; biting to taste. Very toxic. Stimulant, cardiotonic, analgesic, diaphoretic, sedative, alterative, deobstruent, antiarthritic.

Indications: excessive diarrhea, weak pulse, chills, chest and abdominal pain, emphysema, beriberi, adolescent convulsions, fever, nervous disorders, rheumatism, neuralgia, edema, cholera

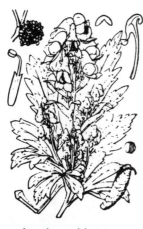

Aconitum chinense

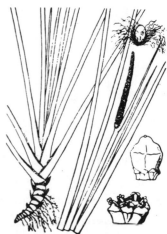

Acorus gramineus

Acorus
(Rock Sweet-flag)

Botanical name: *Acorus gramineus* (Araceae)

Pharmaceutical name: Rhizoma Acori Graminei

Chinese name: *shih-chang-pu* 石菖蒲

From *Shen Nung's Herbal* (superior drug)

Constituents: essential oil, asarone

Properties and actions: warm; pungent. Analgesic, sedative, stomachic, antitoxic, vermifugal.

Indications: mental illness, epilepsy, amnesia, nightmares, diarrhea. Externally applied to carbuncles.

Adenophora

Botanical name: *Adenophora tetraphylla, A. stricta,* or other of the *Adenophora* genus (Campanulaceae)

Pharmaceutical name: Radix Adenophorae

Chinese name: *nan-sha-shen* 南沙参

From *Shen Nung's Herbal*

Constituents: saponin

Properties and actions: slightly cold; sweet yet bitter. Nourishes yin and purifies the lungs, resolves phlegm.

Indications: febrile diseases, thirst, dry mouth, internal heat in the lungs, cough, hemoptysis from coughing

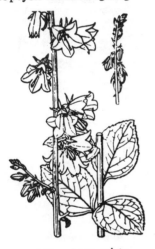

Adenophora stricta

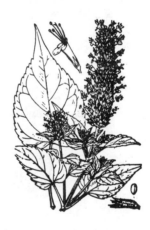

Agastache rugosa

Agastache

Botanical name: *Agastache rugosa* (Labiatae)

Pharmaceutical name: Herba Agastachis

Chinese name: *huo-hsiang* 藿香

From *Chia yu pen tsao* (1061 A.D.)

Constituents: essential oil

Properties and actions: warm, pleasant yet acrid to taste. Clears fevers, resolves moisture, strengthens the stomach and stops vomiting.

Indications: dyspepsia, vomiting with diarrhea, abdominal pain, chest distention due to gastric disorders, the common cold, and headache.

163

Akebia

Botanical name: *Akebia quinata* (Lardizabalaceae)

Pharmaceutical name: Caulis Mutung

Chinese name: *mu-t'ung* 木通

Constituents: akebin, potassium salts

Properties and actions: slightly cold; bitter. Promotes urination, counteracts inflammation and fever, sedates.

Indications: edema, difficult urination, amenorrhea, inadequate lactation

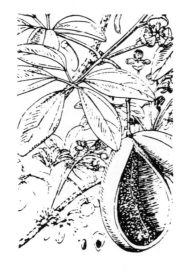

Akebia quinata

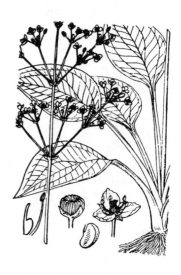

Alisma orientalis

Alisma
(Water Plantain)

Botanical name: *Alisma orientalis, A. plantago-aquatica* (Alismataceae)

Pharmaceutical name: Rhizoma Alismatis

Chinese name: *tse-she, tse-hsieh* 澤舍，澤瀉

Constituents: choline, asparagine, phytosterol, biorin, protein, starch, resin

Properties and actions: bitter. Diuretic, aphrodisiac.

Indications: wet fever, edema, vomiting, diarrhea, gonorrhea, *wu-lin* (five disease conditions involving the urinary tract—kidney stones, polyuria, hematuria, bladder distention, and chyluria)

Aloe

Botanical name: *Aloe barbadensis, A. ferox* (Liliaceae)

Pharmaceutical name: Herba Aloes

Chinese name: *lu-hui* 盧會

Constituents: barbaloin, isobarbaloin, resin, sicaloin, emodin, cinnamic acid, *d*-arabinose, oxydase

Properties and actions: cold; bitter. Anthelmintic, stomachic, laxative.

Indications: children's hernia, epilepsy, constipation. Used externally in conjunction with licorice for eczema.

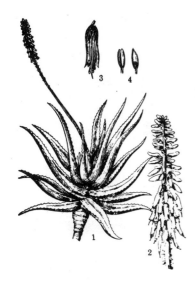

Aloe vera

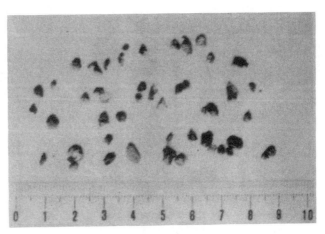

Succinum

Amber (Succinum)
(Fossilized Resin)

Botanical name: *Pinus succinifera* (Pinaceae)

Pharmaceutical name: Succinum—resinous exudate which has been buried a long time and has turned into a clear, fossil-like substance

Chinese name: *hu-po* 琥珀

Properties and actions: bland, sweet. Tonic and alterative.

Indications: epilepsy, insomnia, gonorrhea, hematuria, cuts, contusions, catarrh of the bowels or bladder, convulsive disorders in children

Anemarrhena

Botanical name: *Anemarrhena asphodeloides* (Liliaceae)
Pharmaceutical name: Rhizoma Anemarrhenae
Chinese name: *chih-mu* 知母
Constituents: saponin, asphonin, mucilage, pantothenic acid
Properties and actions: antipyretic, mild carminative
Indications: thirst, cough, urinary and bowel disorders

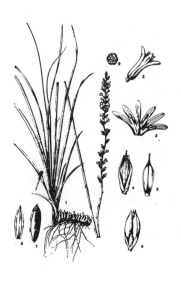

Anemarrhena asphodeloides

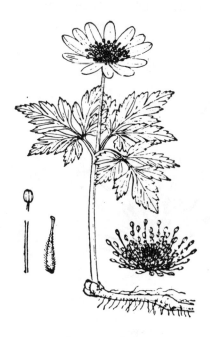

Anemone altaica

Anemone (Altaica)

Botanical name: *Anemone altaica* (Ranunculaceae)

Pharmaceutical name: Rhizoma Anemonis Altaicae

Chinese name: *chiu-chieh-chang-pu* 九節菖蒲

Constituents: saponins, protoanemonin

Properties and actions: stomachic, vermifugal, antitoxic

Indications: fever, diarrhea, nightmares, mental illness, epilepsy. Used externally for carbuncles and scabies.

Angelica

Botanical name: *Angelica dahurica, A. anomala* var. *pai-chi* (Umbelliferae)

Pharmaceutical name: Radix Angelicae Dahuricae

Chinese name: *pai-chih* 白芷

From *The Classic on Mountains and Seas* (400 B.C.)

Constituents: small points of resinous or oily secretion inside

Properties and actions: warm-natured, acrid to taste. Clears the inner organs and dispels gas, warms (excessive) hydration and promotes pus drainage.

Indications: common cold, migraine, dizziness, neuralgia, perspiration

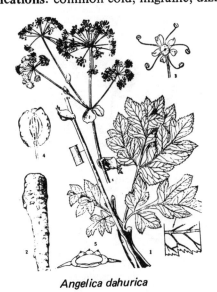

Angelica dahurica

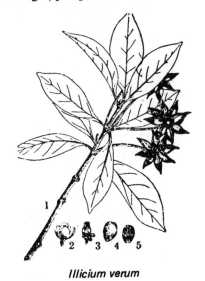

Illicium verum

Anise (Star Anise)
(Chinese Anise)

Botanical name: *Illicium verum* (Magnoliaceae)

Pharmaceutical name: Fructus Anisi Stellati

Chinese name: *pa-chiao-hui-hsiang* 八角茴香

Constituents: essential oil, anethol, caren, methylchavicol, *d*-pinene, cymol, *l*-phellandrene, limonenes, hydroquinone, cineol, furfurol, safrol, farnesol, terpineol, dioxybenzoic acid, anisaldehyde, anisketone

Properties and actions: warm; pungent and sweet

Indications: hernia, chilling pain in the chest, abdominal pain, vomiting, anorexia, cholera, beriberi, constipation, lower back pain, atrophy of the bladder

Apricot

Botanical name: *Prunus armeniaca, P. sibirica, P. mandshurica* (Rosaceae)

Pharmaceutical name: Semen Armeniacae

Chinese name: *hsing-jen* 杏仁

Constituents: amygdalin, hydrocyanic acid

Properties and actions: sour. Antispasmodic, sedative, expectorant.

Indications: sputum, cough, asthma, constipation

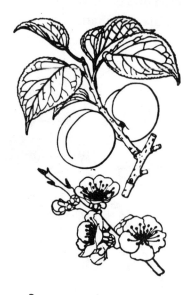

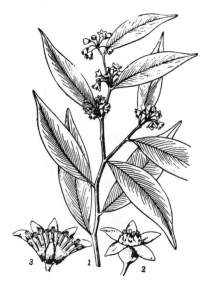

Prunus armeniaca var. *ansu*   *Aquilaria agallocha*

Aquilaria
(Aloes Wood)

Botanical name: *Aquilaria sinensis, A. agallocha* (Thymelaeceae)

Pharmaceutical name: Lignum Aquilariae

Chinese name: *chen-hsiang* 沈香

From *Ming i pieh lu*

Constituents: essential oil, resin

Properties and actions: slightly warm; pungent, sweet and bitter, aromatic. Nutritive, sedative. Reinforces the kidneys, alleviates pain.

Indications: asthma, vomiting, diarrhea, hiccoughs, cardiac and abdominal pain, chills in the waist and knees

Arbor Vitae (Biota)

Botanical name: *Biota orientalis* (Cupressaceae)

Pharmaceutical name: Semen Biotae—dried, ripe seeds

Chinese name: *po-tzu-jen* 柏子仁

From *Shen Nung's Herbal* (superior drug)

Constituents: volatile oils (pinene and caryophyllene), pinipicrin, thujin, tannin, and resin

Properties and actions: bittersweet. Astringent, expectorant, antitussive, nutritive tonic.

Indications: palpitations, insomnia, amnesia, ephidrosis, nocturnal emissions, constipation, expectoration, bronchitis, asthma, dry stools; a delicate constitution

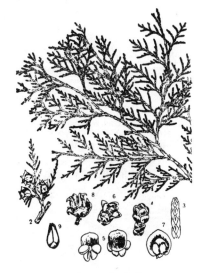

Biota orientalis

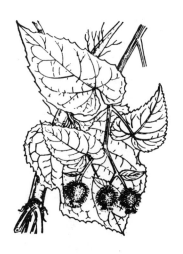

Arctium lappa

Arctium
(Burdock)

Botanical name: *Arctium lappa* (Compositae)

Pharmaceutical name: Fructus Arctii

Chinese name: *niu-pang-tzu* 牛蒡子

Constituents: arctiin, arctigenin, gobosterin, essential oil, fatty oil

Properties and actions: pungent, sweet, mucilaginous, slightly bitter. Diuretic, antipyretic, expectorant, antiphlogistic.

Indications: gout, chills, fever, cough, sore throat, dermatitis, ulcers

Arisaema
(Jack-in-the-Pulpit)

Botanical name: *Arisaema consanquineum, A. amurense* and other varieties of the Araceae family

Pharmaceutical name: Rhizoma Arisaematis

Chinese name: *tien-nan-hsing* 天南星

From *Shen Nung's Herbal* (inferior drug)

Properties and actions: warm; bitter; toxic. Sedative. Relieves spasms and pain, loosens mucus, dispels clots, reduces swelling.

Indications: convulsions in children, monoplegia. Externally used for painful swellings.

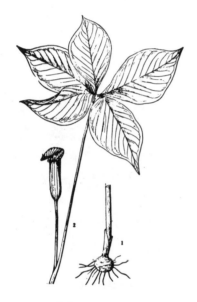

Arisaema amurense

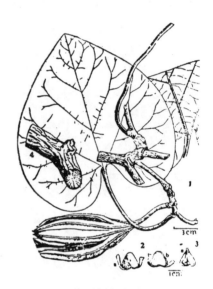

Hocquartia manshuriensis

Aristolochia (Hocquartia)
(Birthwort)

Botanical name: *Aristolochia manshuriensis (Hocquartia manshuriensis)*

Pharmaceutical name: Caulis Aristolochiae

Chinese name: *kuan-mu-t'ung* 關木通

Constituents: aristolochine

Properties and actions: bitter. Antitussive, expectorant.

Indications: asthma, bronchitis

Aristolochia
(Frail Birthwort)

Botanical name: *Aristolochia debilis* (Aristolochiaceae)

Pharmaceutical name: Fructus Aristolochiae

Chinese name: *ma-tou-ling* 馬兜鈴

Constituents: poisonous alkaloid aristolochine

Properties and actions: slightly cold; bitter and pungent. Antitussive, expectorant. Dispels flatus; stimulates *ch'i;* strengthens the stomach; relieves coughing, asthma, and bronchitis.

Indications: flushing up of pulmonary *ch'i,* cough, gasping, fever in the lungs, hemoptysis, hemorrhoids, ascites

Note: Toxic doses caused cardiac and respiratory arrest in experimental animals.

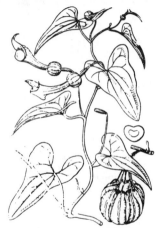

Aristolochia debilis

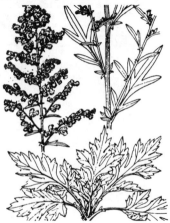

Artemisia vulgaris var. *indica*

Artemisia
(Mugwort or St. John's Plant)

Botanical name: *Artemisia vulgaris* var. *indica* (Compositae)

Pharmaceutical name: Folium Artemisiae

Chinese name: *ai-yeh* 艾葉

Constituents: essential oil (cineol and thujone), tannin, resin, adenine, artemisin, vitamins A, B_1, B_2, C, and D

Properties and actions: slightly warm; bitter, fragrant. Hemostatic, stomachic. Quiets the fetus, dispels gas and "cold."

Indications: abdominal pain, chronic dysentery, hemoptysis, menstrual irregularity, sterility, itching

Artemisia (Capillaris)
(Wormwood)

Botanical name: *Artemisia capillaris* (Compositae)
Pharmaceutical name: Herba Artemisiae
Chinese name: *yin-ch'en-hao* 茵陳蒿
Constituents: β-pinene, capillane, capillene

Properties and actions: slightly cold; bitter. Antipyretic, diuretic.
Indications: sweating fever, jaundice, painful urination

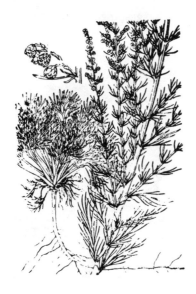

Artemisia capillaris

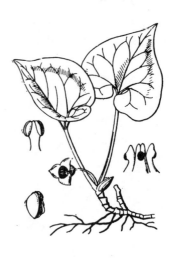

Asarum sieboldi

Asarum
(Wild Ginger)

Botanical name: *Asarum sieboldi* (Aristolochiaceae)
Pharmaceutical name: Herba cum Radice Asari
Chinese name: *pei-hsin, hsi-hsin* 北辛，細辛
Constituents: essential oil methyl, eugenol, phenol, safrol, pinene, encarvone, a sarinine
Properties and actions: neutral; acrid to taste. Analgesic, sedative, expectorant, diuretic.
Indications: nasal problems, toothache, headache, rheumatism, asthma

Aster

Botanical name: *Aster tataricus* (Compositae)

Pharmaceutical name: Radix Asteris

Chinese name: *tzu-wan* 紫菀

From *Shen Nung's Herbal*

Con.tituents: saponins, shionon, quercetin, arabinose

Properties and actions: warm bitter and sweet. Quiets the nervous system. Especiaiiy used to quiet restless, crying children.

Indications: pulmonary conditions—coughing, asthma, pain, hemoptysis; hematuria; dysuria; puerperal heinorrhage

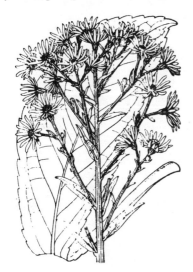

Aster tataricus

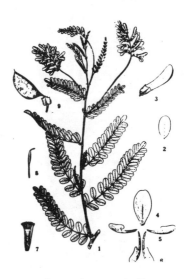

Astragalus mongholicus

Astragalus
(Milk Vetch)

Botanical name: *Astragaius membranaceus, A. mongholicus, A. tongolensis, Hedysarum polyhotrys* (Leguminosae)

Pharmaceutical name: Radix Astragali

Chinese name: *huang-ch'i* 黄耆

Constituents: choline, betaine, amino acid, sucrose

Properties and actions: stops perspiration, strengthens the spleen

Indications: lack of vigor, night sweats

Atractylodes
(Paichu)

Botanical name: *Atractylodes macrocephala, A. lancea, A. ovata, A. japonica* (Compositae)

Pharmaceutical name: Rhizoma Atractylodis

Chinese name: *pai-chu, tsang-chu* 白朮，蒼朮

Constituents: the essential oil atractylone, atractylol

Properties and actions: warm; bitter. Supplements the spleen (general tonic to increase appetite and promote good health), induces perspiration, relieves asthma, promotes diuresis.

Indications: fatigue, anorexia, diarrhea, edema, fever and chills without perspiration

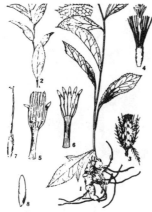

Atractylodes lancea

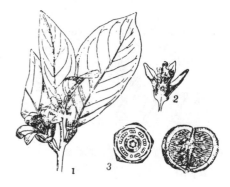

Citrus aurantium

Aurantium (Chih-ko)
(Bitter Orange)

Botanical name: *Citrus aurantium, C. kotokan, C. natsudaidai, C. wilsonii, Poncirus trifoliata* (Rutaceae)

Pharmaceutical name: Fructus Citri Aurantii—almost ripe fruit dried and preserved for several years is preferred

Chinese name: *chih-k'o* 枳殼

From *Shen Nung's Herbal*

Constituents: limonene, linalool, linalyl acetate, methyl anthranilate

Properties and actions: aromatic. Stomachic, diuretic, antidiarrheic.

Indications: excessive sputum, visceral distention, abdominal swelling, indigestion, constipation

Bamboo

Botanical name: *Phyllostachys nigra* var. *henonis* (Gramineae)

Pharmaceutical name: Caulis Bambusae in Taenia—leaves

Chinese name: *chu-ju* 竹茹

From *Shen Nung's Herbal*

Properties and actions: cool; bland. Expectorant, antipyretic, diuretic.

Indications: asthma, cough, hemoptysis, vomiting, nosebleeds, fever due to stress

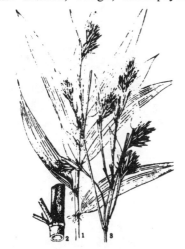

Phyllostachys nigra var. *henonis*

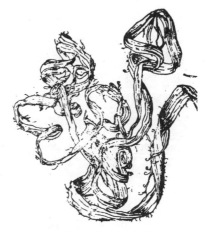

Caulis Bambusae in Taenia

Bamboo
(Bamboo Sap)

Botanical name: *Phyllostachys nigra* var. *henonis* (Gramineae)

Pharmaceutical name: Succus Bambusae—extracted juice of the stem

Chinese name: *chu-li* 竹瀝

From *Pen tsao kang mu*

Properties and actions: antipyretic, antitussive, hemostatic. Removes internal heat, cools.

Indications: cough, thirst

Beeswax (Flava Wax)

Pharmaceutical name: Cera Flava—used for coating pills, base for ointment

Chinese name: *huang-la, feng-la* 黃蠟，蜂蠟

From *Shen Nung's Herbal* (superior drug)

Benincasa
(Chinese Wax Gourd or Winter Melon)

Botanical name: *Benincasa hispida* (Cucurbitaceae)

Pharmaceutical name: Semen Benincasae—dried ripe seeds

Chinese name: *tung-kua-tzu* 冬瓜子

From *Shen Nung's Herbal* (superior drug)

Constituents: urease, adenine, histidine, saponins

Properties and actions: sweet. Anti-inflammative, antitussive, diuretic.

Indications: edema, thirst, intestinal pain, pain in the lungs, cough, suppuration

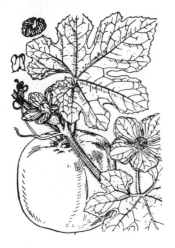

Benincasa hispida

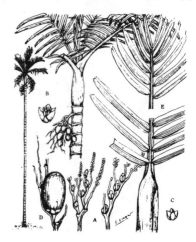

Areca catechu

Betel Nut
(Areca)

Botanical name: *Areca catechu* (Palmae)

Pharmaceutical name: Semen Arecae; Pericarpium Arecae

Chinese name: *pin-lang; ta-fu-pi* 檳榔；大腹皮

Constituents: palmitic, oleic, stearic, caproic, caprylic, lauric, myristic acids; mannosan; galactans; tannin; choline; arecoline; arecaidine; guvacoline; guvacine

Properties and actions: warm; pungent. Stimulates peristalsis; a bronchial constrictory and vermicidal. Stimulates *ch'i.*

Indications: intestinal parasites, chest pain and distention, abdominal pain, dysentery, malaria, edema, beriberi

Remarks: Side effects may be mild dyspnea, diaphoresis, vertigo, and nausea.

Black Pepper

Botanical name: *Piper nigrum* (Piperaceae)

Pharmaceutical name: Fructus Piperis Album

Chinese name: *hu-chiao* 胡椒

Constituents: piperine, piperidine, chavicine, volatile oils (*l*-phellandrene and caryo-phyllene)

Properties and actions: hot; pungent. Carminative, stomachic. Warms and aids elimination.

Indications: stagnancy of chilling and wetness, *ch'i* stagnancy in the chest, sputum, diarrhea, pyrosis

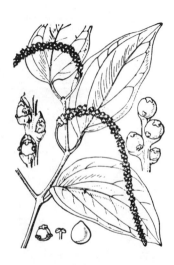

Piper nigrum

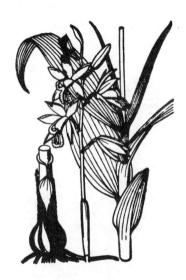

Bletilla striata

Bletilla

Botanical name: *Bletilla striata* (Orchidaceae)

Pharmaceutical name: Tuber Bletillae. Fresh tubers are dried in the sun.

Chinese name: *pai-chi* 白及

From *Shen Nung's Herbal*

Constituents: mucilage, essential oil, glycogen

Properties and actions: bland and bitter. Emollient.

Indications: hemoptysis, nosebleeds, knife wounds, carbuncles, burns, dysentery, hemorrhoids, ague. Childhood diseases in a boy or girl of a dyspeptic nature.

Bupleurum
(Hare's Ear)

Botanical name: *Bupleurum chinense, B. scorzonerae-folium, B. falcatum* (Umbelliferae)

Pharmaceutical name: Radix Bupleuri

Chinese name: *ch'ai-hu* 柴胡

Constituents: palmitic acid, stearic acid, linolic acid, spinasterol, stigmasterol, adonitol, saponins

Properties and actions: cold; bitter to taste. Antipyretic, diaphoretic. Neutralizes the liver, regulates menstruation.

Indications: alternating fever, swollen throat, bitter taste, deafness, vertigo, vomiting, malaria, irregular menstruation

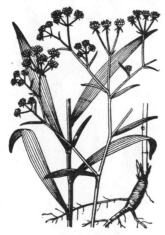

Bupleurum falcatum

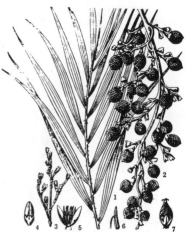

Calamus draco

Calamus
(Dragon Blood)

Botanical name: *Calamus draco* (Palmae)

Pharmaceutical name: Sanguis Draconis—decocted and compressed resin from the fruit and trunk

Chinese name: *hsieh-chieh* 血竭

Properties and actions: bland, sweet and salty. Promotes tissue granulation, stimulates blood circulation, alleviates pain. Externally used to stop bleeding and promote healing.

Indications: pain in the heart and abdomen, knife wounds, wounds, contusions

178

Cannabis
(Hemp)

Botanical name: *Cannabis sativa* (Cannabinaceae)

Pharmaceutical name: Semen Cannabis—seeds

Chinese name: *ta-ma-jen* 大麻仁

From *Shen Nung's Herbal*

Constituents: protein, lipids, choline, trigonelline, xylose, inositol, phytin, enzymes (lipase, maltase, emulsin, linamarase, amylase, urease, nuclease, erepsin, tryptase, catalase)

Properties and actions: sweet, aromatic. Nutritive tonic, vermifuge, emollient.

Indications: constipation, intestinal heat

Note: Presently, this herb has been substituted by *Linum usitatissimum* L.

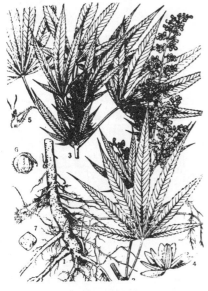

Cannabis sativa

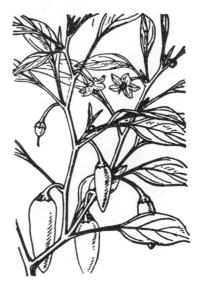

Capsicum annum

Capsicum
(Red Pepper or Chili)

Botanical name: *Capsicum annum* (Solanaceae)

Pharmaceutical name: Fructus Capsici

Chinese name: *la-chiao* 辣椒

Properties and actions: a stimulant, counterirritant, stomachic. Promotes sweating.

Indications: rheumatism

Cardamon

Botanical name: *Amomum cardamomum* (Zingiberaceae)
Pharmaceutical name: Fructus Amomi Cardamomi
Chinese name: *pai-tou-kou* 白豆蔻
From *Ming-i-pieh-lu*
Constituents: essential oil comprising cineol, camphor, *d*-borneol, terpineol
Properties and actions: pungent, slightly bitter, aromatic. Stomachic, antiemetic.
Indications: stomachache, abdominal distention, gastric upset, belching, hiccoughs, drunkenness

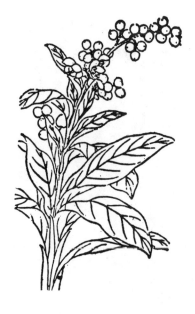

Amomum cardamomum

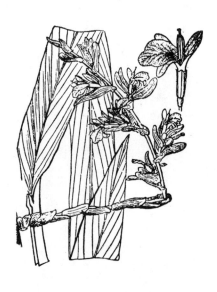

Elettaria cardamomum

Cardamon (Elettaria)

Botanical name: *Elettaria cardamomum* (Zingiberaceae)
Pharmaceutical name: Fructus Cardamomi
Chinese name: *hsiao-tou-kou* 小豆蔻
Properties and actions: aromatic; carminative. Condiment, spice.

Cardamon, Chinese
(Bastard Cardamon)

Botanical name: *Amomum villosum, A. xanthioides, A. chinense* (Zingiberaceae)

Pharmaceutical name: Fructus et Semen Amomi

Chinese name: *sha-jen, sha-jen-k'o, sha-k'o* 砂仁，砂仁殼，砂殼

Constituents: essential oil (*d*-camphor, linalool, borneol, nerolidol), fat, carbohydrate

Properties and actions: treats abdominal pain and distention, gastric disorders

Indications: poor digestion, cramps, gas, hiccoughs, vomiting, diarrhea, dysentery

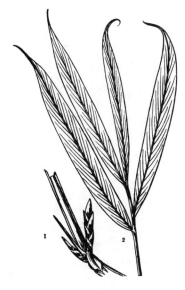

Amomum xanthioides

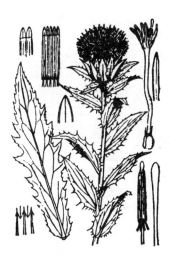

Carthamus tinctorius

Carthamus

Botanical name: *Carthamus tinctorius* L. (Compositae)

Pharmaceutical name: Flos Carthami

Chinese name: *hung-hua* 紅花

From *Kai pao pen tsao* (973 A.D.)

Constituents: carthamic acid, safflower yellow.

Properties and actions: warm, acrid to taste. Resolves bruises and stimulates tissue regeneration. Activates and clears meridian channels.

Indications: gynecological disorders such as amenorrhea, dystocia, hemorrhage after childbirth, and stagnant blood

Cassia
(Senna)

Botanical name: *Cassia angustifolia* (Leguminosae)

Pharmaceutical name: Folium Sennae

Chinese name: *fan-hsieh-yeh* 番瀉葉

Constituents: rhein, aloe-emodin, glycosides, sennoside A and B, sennacrol, sennapicrin, sennarhamnetin, kaempferol, kaempferin, volatile oil

Properties and actions: cold; bittersweet. Leaflets and pods are used as a purgative. Eliminates stagnancy, smooths bowel movements.

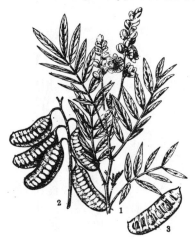

Cassia angustifolia

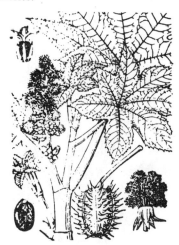

Ricinus communis

Castor Oil Plant (Ricinus)

Botanical name: *Ricinus communis* (Euphorbiaceae)

Pharmaceutical name: Semen Ricini

Chinese name: *pi-ma-tzu* 蓖麻子

Constituents: castor oil, albumin ricin, toxic alkaloid ricinine

Properties and actions: bland, sweet and pungent. Draws out pus, stops pain, relieves constipation, corrects prolapses.

Indications: vapor distention, difficult urination, intestinal stagnancy. Used externally for carbuncles, furunculosis, scabies, scrofula, edematous toxin, throat paralysis, drooping eyes and mouth.

Note: Ingestion of the seeds may cause violent gastroenteritis with nausea, headache, persistent vomiting, colic, thirst, emaciation, and great debility.

Catechu

Botanical name: *Acacia catechu* (Leguminosae)

Pharmaceutical name: Catechu

Chinese name: *erh-cha* 兒茶

From *Pen ts'ao kang mu*

Properties and actions: hemostatic and expectorant. Cools and astringes.

Indications: stomatitis, moist abscesses, hemorrhoidal swelling, fever and cough

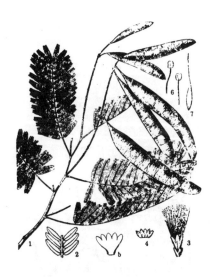

Acacia catechu

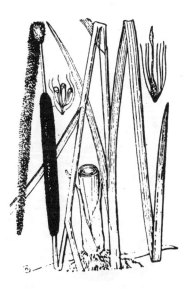

Typha angustata

Cattail (Typha)

Botanical name: *Typha angustifolia* (Typhaceae)

Pharmaceutical name: Pollen Typhae—dried pollen

Chinese name: *pu-huang* 蒲黃

From *Shen Nung's Herbal*

Constituents: iso-rhamnetin, fatty oil, a sitosterol

Properties and actions: bland and sweet. A hemostatic if fried until charred, diuretic.

Indications: prolonged menstruation, aching arms after childbirth, pain in the heart and abdomen, oliguria, bloody urine, contusions

Chain Fern (Cibotium)

Botanical name: *Cibotium barometz* (Cyatheaceae)

Pharmaceutical name: Rhizoma Cibotii—dried rhizomes

Chinese name: *kou-chi* 狗脊

From *Shen Nung's Herbal*

Properties and actions: warm; bitter and sweet. Strengthens the spine; stimulates the liver, kidneys, and male reproductive organs. Good for old men.

Indications: chills caused by wind, rheumatism, lower back pain, weak feet, urinary incontinence, cloudy urine

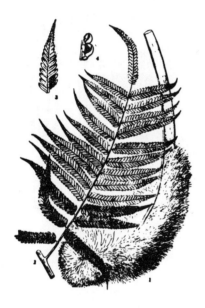

Cibotium barometz

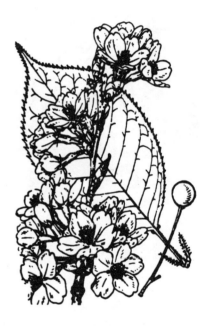

Prunus yedoensis

Cherry

Botanical name: *Prunus yedoensis* (Rosaceae)

Pharmaceutical name: Cortex Pruni

Chinese name: *ying-pi* 櫻皮

Constituents: sakuranin

Properties and actions: astringent, antiphlogistic. Used as a cough syrup.

Chianghuo

Botanical name: *Notopterygium incisium* (Umbelliferae)

Pharmaceutical name: Rhizoma Notopterygii—dried roots and tubers

Chinese name: *ch'iang-huo* 羌活

From *Shen Nung's Herbal*

Properties and actions: diaphoretic, carminative, analgesic

Indications: common cold, headache, generalized discomfort, severe chills, fever without sweating, rheumatic neuralgia, swollen carbuncles, sloughing ulcers, injuries

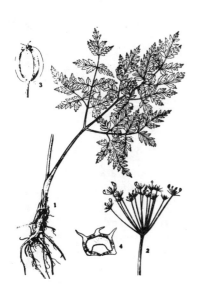

Notopterygium incisium

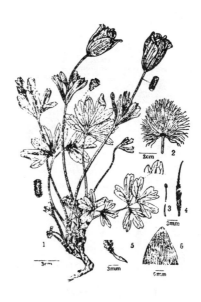

Pulsatilla chinensis

Chinese Anemone

Botanical name: *Pulsatilla chinensis* (Ranunculaceae)

Note: *Pulsatilla chinensis = Anemone chinensis*

Pharmaceutical name: Radix Pulsatillae Chinensis

Chinese name: *pai-tou-weng* 白頭翁

From *Shen Nung's Herbal*

Properties and actions: cool; bitter taste. Eliminates fever, cools the blood.

Indications: fever toxin, bloody diarrhea, nosebleeds, warm malaria

Chinese Clematis

Botanical name: *Clematis chinensis* (Ranunculaceae)
Pharmaceutical name: Radix Clematidis
Chinese name: *wei-ling-hsien* 威靈仙

From *Kai pao pen tsao*
Constituents: anemonin
Properties and actions: warm; bitter and pungent. Dispels flatus, removes moisture, alleviates pain.
Indications: rheumatic pain; jaundice; edema; pain at the waist, knees, arms, and legs

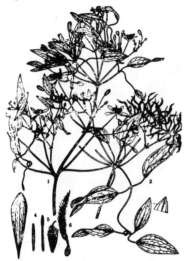 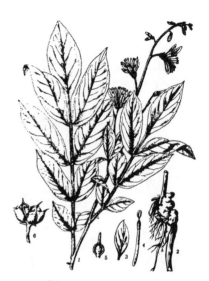

Clematis chinensis   *Dictamnus dasycarpus*

Chinese Dittany (Fraxinella)

Botanical name: *Dictamnus dasycarpus* (Rutaceae)
Pharmaceutical name: Radicis Cortex Dictamni
Chinese name: *pai-hsien-p'i* 白鮮皮
From *Shen Nung's Herbal*
Constituents: alkaloid dictamnine
Properties and actions: cool; bitter taste. Eliminates wet fevers, relieves rheumatism, regulates urination, loosens stiff joints.
Indications: "wind" paralysis, wet boils, jaundice, scabies, eczema, impetigo
Conformation: weakness and chilling in the lower warmer

Chinese Quince (Chaenomeles)

Botanical name: *Chaenomeles lagenaria* (Rosaceae)

Pharmaceutical name: Fructus Chaenomelis—dried ripe fruit

Chinese name: *mu-kua* 木瓜

From *Ming i pieh lu*

Constituents: vitamin C; malic, tartaric, and citric acids; sometimes hydrocyanic acid

Properties and actions: warm; sour and biting. Dispels internal heat in the liver, improves gastric function, removes moisture, relaxes muscles.

Indications: beriberi, swelling, moist spasms, persistent cough

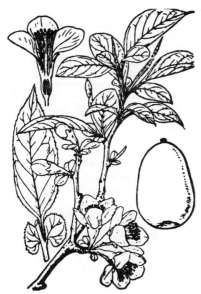

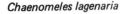

Chaenomeles lagenaria

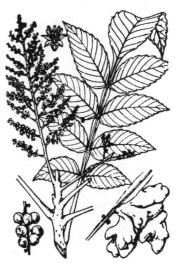

Rhus javanica

Chinese Sumac
(Gallnut)

Botanical name: *Rhus javanica* (Anacardiaceae)

Pharmaceutical name: Galla Rhi Chinensis et Potaninii—gall from the leaves or leaf-stalks caused by an insect, usually an aphid

Chinese name: *wu-pei-tzu* 五倍子

Properties and actions: bland and sour. Astringent and hemostatic.

Indications: pulmonary weakness, cough, prolonged diarrhea, anal prolapse, excessive sweating, melena, cuts

187

Chrysanthemum

Botanical name: *Chrysanthemum indicum* (Compositae)

Pharmaceutical name: Flos Chrysanthemi

Chinese name: *chu-hua* 菊花

From *Shen Nung's Herbal* (superior drug)

Constituents: essential oil, adenine, choline, stachydrine

Properties and actions: slightly *han* (cold) properties, bitter yet pleasant to taste. Carminative, antipyretic, and detoxifying.

Indications: vertigo, ophthalmia with swelling and pain, headache with fever

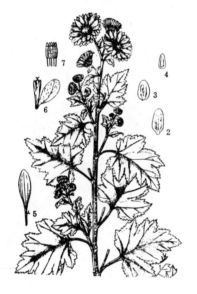

Chrysanthemum morifolium

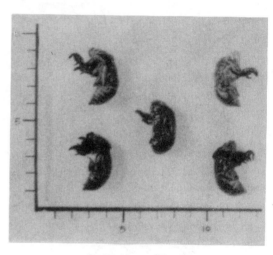

Periostracum Cicadae

Cicada

Scientific name: *Cryptotmypana atrata*

Pharmaceutical name: Periostracum Cicadae

Chinese name: *ch'an-shui* 蟬蛻

Properties and actions: disperses heat, stabilizes pulmonary functions, stops convulsions

Indications: gout, fever, headache, impaired vocal function, coughing, sore throat, measles, infantile nocturnal crying, tetanus

Cimicifuga
(Bugbane)

Botanical name: *Cimicifuga foetida, C. dahurica, C. simplex* (Ranunculaceae)
Pharmaceutical name: Rhizoma Cimicifugae
Chinese name: *sheng-ma* 升麻

Constituents: tannin, the resin cimicifugin, cimicifugenol
Properties and actions: slightly cold; bitter. Stomachic, antipyretic, sedative, analgesic.
Indications: intoxication, headache, chills, fever, sore throat, canker sores, chronic diarrhea, dysentery, rectocele, rashes, measles, smallpox, erysipelas, uterine prolapse

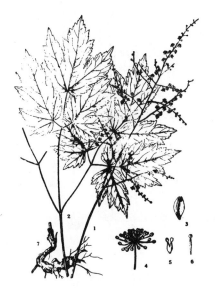

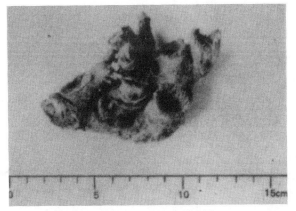

Rhizoma Cimicifugae

Cimicifuga dahurica

Cinnabar

Pharmaceutical name: Cinnabaris, red mercuric sulfide (HgS)
Chinese name: *chu-sha* 朱砂
From *Shen Nung's Herbal* (superior drug)
Properties and actions: slightly cold; sweet. Poisonous. Sedative and antitoxic. Settles nerves and controls convulsions, detoxifies.
Indications: epileptic seizures, palpitations due to fear, insomnia, nightmares. Externally applied on carbuncles, scabies, and painful swelling in the throat.

Cinnamon

Botanical name: *Cinnamomum cassia* (Lauraceae)

Pharmaceutical name: Cortex et Ramulus Cinnamomi

Chinese name: *kuei-p'i, kuei-chih* 桂皮，桂枝

Constituents: ash, caoxalate, starch, tannin, essential oil, cinnamic aldehyde, furfurol, cinnamic acid, cinnamyl acetate, terpene

Properties and actions: very hot; pleasant, yet acrid to taste. Antitussive, carminative. Regulates pulse, promotes sweating, relaxes muscles, stimulates appetite.

Indications: colds, typhoid fever, headache, external weakness, cough, rheumatic pain, pulmonary malfunction, gout

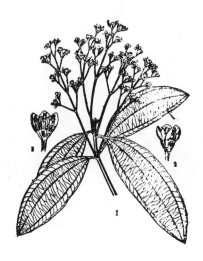

Cinnamomum cassia

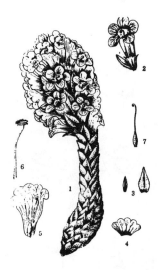

Cistanche salsa

Cistanche
(Broomrape)

Botanical name: *Cistanche salsa* (Orobanchaceae)

Pharmaceutical name: Herba Cistanches—dried stems and leaves

Chinese name: *jou-tsung-jung* 肉蓯蓉

From *Shen Nung's Herbal* (superior drug)

Properties and actions: nutritive, tonic, aphrodisiac

Indications: impotence, infertility, constipation, anemia, chills and pain in the waist and knees

Cloves

Botanical name: *Eugenia caryophyllata* (Myrtaceae)

Pharmaceutical name: Flos Caryophylli—dried floral buds

Chinese name: *ting-hsiang* 丁香

Constituents: volatile oils eugenol, acetyl-eugenol, caryophyllene, furfural, vanillin, methylamylketone

Properties and actions: warm; pungent. Antiseptic, antispasmodic, stomachic, carminative. Warms the body, alleviates pain, increases circulation.

Indications: hiccoughs, vomiting, diarrhea, stomachache, abdominal pain

Contraindications: febrile diseases, yin weakness, inside fever, gastrosia, acute gastroenteritis, gastrorrhagia

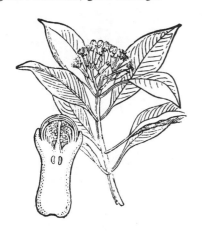

Eugenia caryophyllata

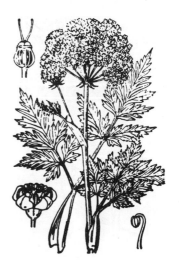

Cnidium officinale

Cnidium
(Szechuan Lovage)

Botanical name: *Cnidium officinale, Ligusticum wallichii* (Umbelliferae)

Pharmaceutical name: Rhizoma Cnidii

Chinese name: *ch'uan-hsiung* 川芎

Constituents: ferulic acid, cnidium lactone, ligustilide, butyphthalide

Properties and actions: analgesic. Stimulates blood circulation, lowers blood pressure, induces uterine contraction, stops bleeding after childbirth.

Indications: headache, abdominal pain, convulsions, diarrhea, suppressed and irregular menstruation

Coix
(Job's Tears)

Botanical name: *Coix lachryma-jobi* (Gramineae)

Pharmaceutical name: Semen Coicis

Chinese name: *i-i-jen, i-mi-jen, i-yi-jen* 薏苡仁，薏米仁

Constituents: starch; fat; sterol; vitamin B; protein; amino acids leucine, tyrosine, lycine, glutamic acid, arginine, histidine

Properties and actions: slightly cold; bland to taste. Nutritive, refrigerant, diuretic.

Indications: fever, edema, beriberi, diarrhea, muscular spasms, intestinal pain, pulmonary disorders, leukorrhea, rheumatoid arthritis, difficult urination

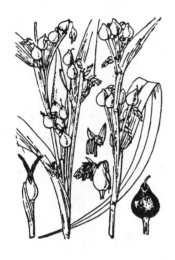

Coix lachryma-jobi

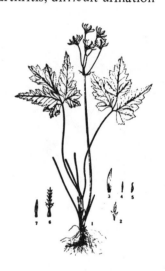

Coptis chinensis

Coptis
(Goldenthread)

Botanical name: *Coptis chinensis, C. japonica, C. tectoides, C. teeta* (Ranunculaceae)

Pharmaceutical name: Rhizoma Coptidis

Chinese name: *huang-lien, chi-lien* 黄連

Constituents: alkaloids coptisine, worenine, berberine

Properties and actions: cold; bitter. Stomachic, digestive, antidysenteric, antipyretic.

Indications: fever, toxins, moisture, heart distress, thirst, dysentery, abdominal pain, hemoptysis, ophthalmia, canker sores, scabies

Cordyceps

Botanical name: *Cordyceps sinensis* (Clavicipitaceae)

Pharmaceutical name: Sclerotium Cordycipitis Sinensis—dried fungus which grows
on the pupae of the Lepidoptera family

Chinese name: *tung-chung-hsia-tsao* 冬蟲夏草

Properties and actions: warm; sweet. Restorative and tonic.

Indications: weakness, fatigue, cough, bloody sputum, phthisis, pain in the lower
back and knees, spermatorrhea, jaundice, impotence, serious injuries

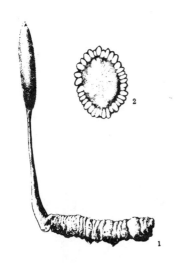

Cordyceps sinensis

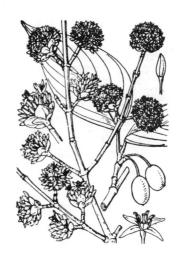

Cornus officinalis

Cornus
(Asiatic Cornelian Cherry)

Botanical name: *Cornus officinalis* (Cornaceae)

Pharmaceutical name: Fructus Corni

Chinese name: *shan-chu-yu* 山茱萸

Constituents: cornin, tannin, resin, tartaric acid

Properties and actions: slightly warm; sour and bitter. Antipyretic, astringent tonic.
Supplements liver and kidneys.

Indications: liver and kidney disorders, tinnitus, nocturnal emission, impotence,
frequent urination

Corydalis

Botanical name: *Corydalis bulbosa, C. ambigua, C. nakai, C. remota* (Papaveraceae)

Pharmaceutical name: Tuber Corydalis

Chinese name: *yen-hu-suo, hsuan-hu* 延胡索，玄胡

Constituents: corydaline A to K, 11 alkaloids, protopine, berberine, tetrahydrop-almitine

Properties and actions: warm; acrid, bitter. Relieves pain, stimulates energy production and blood circulation.

Indications: cardiac, abdominal, flank, and knee pain; injuries from falling; extravasated blood; menstrual irregularity

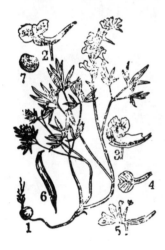

Corydalis bulbosa

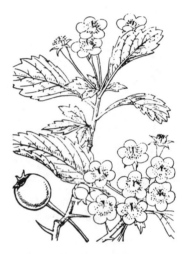

Crataegus cuneata

Crataegus
(Red Haw or Hawthorn)

Botanical name: *Crataegus cuneata, C. pinnatifida* (Rosaceae)

Pharmaceutical name: Fructus Crataegi

Chinese name: *shan-cha* 山楂

Constituents: protein, carbohydrate, fat, citric acid, vitamin C

Properties and actions: warm; sweet and sour. Laxative, stomachic, deobstruent, alterative. Prevents scurvy.

Indications: food stagnancy, hardening and distention in the chest and abdomen, hernia, menorrhagia, aching arms after childbirth

Croton

Botanical name: *Croton tiglium* (Euphorbiaceae)

Pharmaceutical name: Semen Tiglii

Chinese name: *pa-tou* 巴豆

Constituents: croton oil, resin, glyceride of tiglic acid, crotin

Properties and actions: hot; pungent. Poisonous. Violent purgative.

Indications: chilling stagnancy, sputum, edema, dysentery, obstinate diarrhea, delayed menstruation, tumors, ranula (cystic tumor beneath the tongue), apoplexy, paralysis, toothache, throat ailments

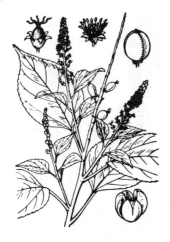
Croton tiglium

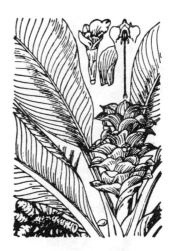
Curcuma longa

Curcuma
(Tumeric)

Botanical name: *Curcuma longa* (Zingiberaceae)

Pharmaceutical name: Rhizoma Curcumae Longae

Chinese name: *chiang-huang* 薑黃

Constituents: essential oils turmerol, curcumon, phellandrene, valeric and caproic acids; curcumin

Properties and actions: warm; bitter, pungent, aromatic. Stomachic, cholagogue, hemostatic. Stimulates the gallbladder.

Indications: hemorrhages, dysmenorrhea, abdominal distention, pain in the chest and abdomen, paralysis due to the wind, wounds

Cynanchum

Botanical name: *Cynanchum atratum* (Asclepiadaceae)
Pharmaceutical name: Radix Cynanchi Atrati—the dried root
Chinese name: *pai-wei* 白薇
From *Shen Nung's Herbal*
Constituents: cynanchin
Properties and actions: cool; bitter and salty. Cleans blood fever, renders diuresis.
Indications: fever; scorching fever; diseases of the urinary tract, especially incontinence
Conformation: yin weakness, fever due to "wind"

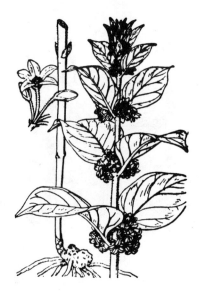

Cynanchum atratum

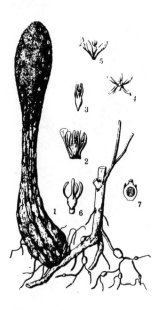

Cynomorium coccineum

Cynomorium

Botanical name: *Cynomorium coccineum* (Cynomoriaceae)
Pharmaceutical name: Herba Cynomorii
Chinese name: *suo-yang* 鎖陽
From *Pen tsao tsung hsin*
Constituents: enzyme, fatty oil, sugar
Properties and actions: warm; sweet. Nutritive, tonic, aphrodisiac, spermatopoietic. Strengthens kidneys and male gonads, moisturizes dryness.
Indications: impotence, infertility, weak waist and knees, constipation

Cyperus
(Nut Grass)

Botanical name: *Cyperus rotundus* (Cyperaceae)

Pharmaceutical name: Rhizoma Cyperi

Chinese name: *hsiang-fu-tzu* 香附子

Constituents: sesquiterpenes, essential oil, fat

Properties and actions: slightly bitter, acrid, fragrant. Relieves melancholia and cardiac pain, corrects *ch'i* circulation, relieves congestion, regulates menstrual cycle, alleviates pain, relieves distention.

Indications: stomachache, menstrual irregularity, chest and side pain, nausea and vomiting, traumatic injuries

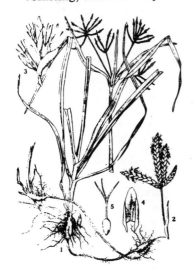

Cyperus rotundus

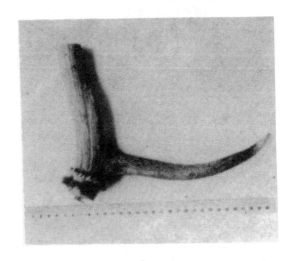

Cornu Cervi

Deer Horn

Pharmaceutical name: Cornu Cervi

Chinese name: *lu-chiao* 鹿角

Constituents: protein, calcium, phosphate, ammonium carbonate, collagen, cartilage

Properties and actions: sweet, pungent, and salty. Antispasmodic, antipyretic, tonic, stimulant.

Indications: phthisis; pain in the flank, lower abdomen and spine; abscess; ulcers; carbuncles

Dendrobium

Botanical name: *Dendrobium nobile* (Orchidaceae)
Pharmaceutical name: Herba Dendrobii
Chinese name: *shih-hu* 石斛
From *Shen Nung's Herbal* (superior drug)
Constituents: dendrobine
Properties and actions: cold; sweet and light, slightly salty. Nutritive, salivant, stomachic. Nourishes yin and promotes salivation.
Indications: fever, thirst from stress, mild fever following an illness

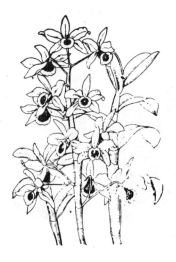

Dendrobium nobile

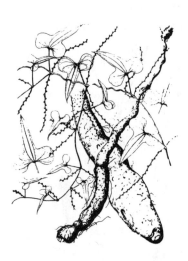

Dioscorea doryophora

Dioscorea
(Yam)

Botanical name: *Dioscorea batatas, D. alata, D. doryophora* (Dioscoreaceae)
Pharmaceutical name: Rhizoma Dioscoreae
Chinese name: *shan-yao* 山藥
Constituents: starch, mucilage, amylase, albuminoid matter, fat, sugar, amino acids (arginine, leucine, tyrosine), glutamine
Properties and actions: neutral; sweet. Nutrient tonic, digestant.
Indications: diarrhea, dysentery, cough, thirst, nocturnal emission, polyuria

Dipsacus
(Japanese Teasel)

Botanical name: *Dipsacus asper* (Dipsacaceae)

Pharmaceutical name: Radix Dipsaci

Chinese name: *hsu-tuan* 續斷

From *Shen Nung's Herbal*

Constituents: essential oil, alkaloid lamine

Properties and actions: slightly warm; bitter and pungent. Tonic, analgesic, hemostatic. Promotes blood circulation, suppresses uterine contractions.

Indications: painful, inflamed, and swollen carbuncles; premature labor; rheumatoid arthralgia; traumatic injuries

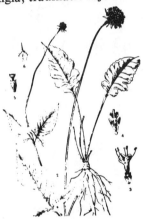

Dipsacus asper

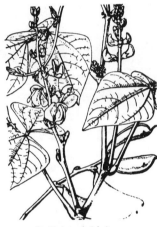

Dolichos lablab

Dolichos
(Hyacinth Bean or Egyptian Kidney Bean)

Botanical name: *Dolichos lablab* (Leguminosae)

Pharmaceutical name: Semen Dolichoris

Chinese name: *pien-tou* 扁豆

From *Ming-i-pieh-lu*

Constituents: protein, fat, ash, emulsin, allantoinase, vitamin C, carbohydrates, calcium, phosphorus, iron

Properties and actions: warm; sweet. A nutritive tonic. Purgative, antitoxic. Arrests diarrhea and vomiting.

Indications: weak spleen and stomach, stagnant internal heat, abdominal distention, leukorrhea, alcoholism

Dragon Bone

Pharmaceutical name: Os Draconis—fossilized bones of dinosaurs and other reptiles

Chinese name: *lung-ku* 龍骨

Constituents: calcium carbonate, calcium phosphate

Actions: sedative

Indications: anxiety, nightmares, nocturnal emissions, sweating, leukorrhea, rectocele, hemoptysis, umbilical abscess, scrotal ulcers, itching

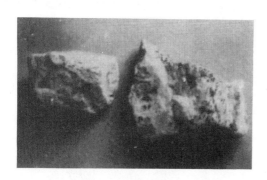

Os Draconis

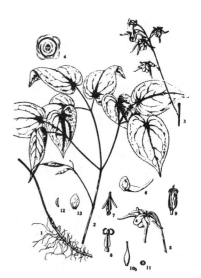

Epimedium macranthum

Epimedium

Botanical name: *Epimedium macranthum, E. grandiflorum* (Berberidaceae)

Pharmaceutical name: Herba Epimedii

Chinese name: *yin-yang-huo* 淫羊藿

From *Shen Nung's Herbal*

Constituents: glycoside (icariin or epimedin), an alkaloid

Properties and actions: warm; sweet. Aphrodisiac. Warms the kidneys, strengthens yang, removes excess moisture and flatulence.

Indications: impotence, weakness and atrophy of the lower back and knees, rheumatism, spasms, numbness of the extremeties, corneal disorders and ulceration of the eye following skin eruptions or rashes

Eriobotrya
(Loquat)

Botanical name: *Eriobotrya japonica* (Rosaceae)

Pharmaceutical name: Folium Eriobotryae

Chinese name: *pi-pa-yeh* 枇杷葉

From *Ming i pieh lu* (general drug)

Constituents: The young leaves contain saponins; the seeds contain amygdalin, hydrocyanic acid, and saponins.

Properties and actions: neutral, bitter to taste. Neutralizes stomach, lowers (excess) energy, quiets coughs, and resolves phlegm.

Indications: cough, expectoration with fever, internal heat in the stomach, vomiting, dysuria, thirst

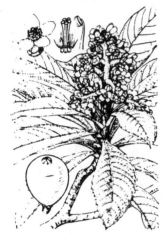

Eriobotryá japonica

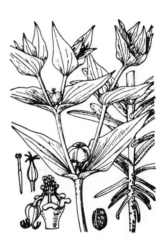

Euphorbia lathyris

Euphorbia (Lathyris)
(Caper Spurge or Mole Plant)

Botanical name: *Euphorbia lathyris* (Euphorbiaceae)

Pharmaceutical name: Semen Euphorbiae Lathyridis

Chinese name: *chien-chin-tzu* 千金子

Constituents: euphorbium, alkaloids

Properties and actions: warm; pungent and bitter. Poisonous. Purgative, diuretic.

Indications: edema, distention, stagnant sputum, prolonged menstruation, food stagnancy. Used externally for ulcerated sores, throat gangrene, and skin diseases.

Evodia

Botanical name: *Evodia rutaecarpa* (Rutaceae)

Pharmaceutical name: Fructus Evodiae

Chinese name: *wu-chu-yu* 吳茱萸

Constituents: alkaloids evodiamine and rutaecarpine

Properties and actions: bitter and pungent. Muscle stimulant (especially of the uterus), central nerve stimulant, carminative. Increases blood pressure.

Indications: chills, melancholy, nausea, headache, chest and abdominal pain, vomiting, diarrhea, beriberi, edema, abscess of mouth and tongue

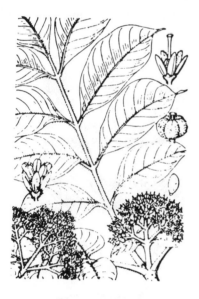

Evodia rutaecarpa

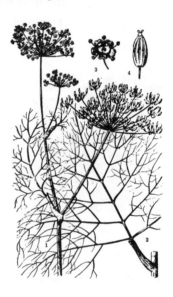

Foeniculum vulgare

Fennel

Botanical name: *Foeniculum vulgare* (Umbelliferae)

Pharmaceutical name: Fructus Foeniculi

Chinese name: *hsiao-hui-hsiang, hui-hsiang* 小茴香，茴香

Constituents: essential oil, fatty oil, starch, sugars, protein

Properties and actions: sharp and sweet. Stomachic. Relieves chills, abdominal distention, vomiting, and diarrhea; promotes digestion; resolves phlegm; stimulates milk production.

Indications: hernia, stomachache, indigestion, abdominal distention, vomiting

Flax (Sesame)
(Linseed)

Botanical name: *Linum usitatissimum* (Linnaceae)

Pharmaceutical name: Semen Lini

Chinese name: *ya-ma-jen* 亞麻仁

Constituents: proteins, mucilage, fatty oil, linolic acid, linamarin, vitamins A and B$_2$

Properties and actions: warm; sweet. Demulcent, emollient, laxative.

Indications: weakness during convalescence, vertigo, dry intestines, constipation

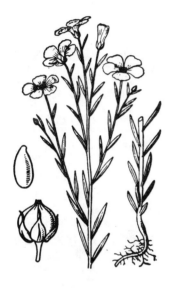

Linum usitatissimum

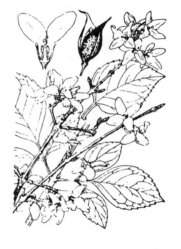

Forsythia suspensa

Forsythia
(Golden Bells)

Botanical name: *Forsythia suspensa* (Oleaceae)

Pharmaceutical name: Fructus Forsythiae

Chinese name: *lien-ch'iao* 連翹

Constituents: quercitrin, rutin, forsythin, phillyrin, saponins

Properties and actions: slightly cold; bitter. Relieves heat, swelling, and suppuration; promotes drainage and diuresis.

Indications: moderate fever, scrofula, erysipelas, eruptions, influenza

Fritillary

Botanical name: *Fritillaria thunbergii* (Liliaceae)

Pharmaceutical name: Bulbus Fritillariae

Chinese name: *pei-mu* 貝母

From *Shen Nung's Herbal* (superior drug)

Constituents: fritilline, verticine

Properties and actions: cold; bitter. Clears fevers, moisturizes the lungs, resolves phlegm, loosens congestion.

Indications: internal heat in the lungs, cough, expectoration, lung disorders

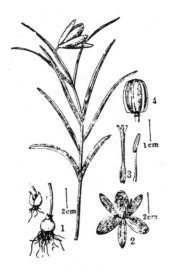

Fritillaria roylei

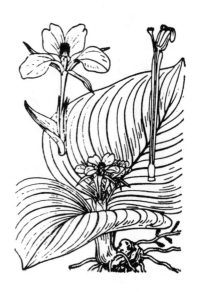

Kaempferia galanga

Galangal

Botanical name: *Kaempferia galanga* (Zingiberaceae)

Pharmaceutical name: Rhizoma Kaempferiae—dried rhizomes

Chinese name: *shan-nai* 山柰

Constituents: essential oil comprising borneol, camphor, cineol, and ethyl alcohol

Properties and actions: warm; pungent, fragrant. Stomachic, carminative, stimulant. Eliminates dandruff or head scabs.

Indications: chilling pain in the chest and abdomen, cold wetness, cholera, toothache

Gambir

Botanical name: *Uncaria rhynchophylla* (Rubiaceae)

Pharmaceutical name: Ramulus et Uncus Uncariae

Chinese name: *kou-teng, tiao-teng* 鈎藤，釣藤

From *Ming i pieh lu* (inferior drug)

Constituents: the alkaloid rhynchophylline

Properties and actions: cold, pleasant yet slightly bitter to taste. Clears fevers, soothes the liver, stops gas (flatus) formation, relieves convulsions.

Indications: infantile febrile diseases, vertigo, hypertension with headache, and epilepsy in children

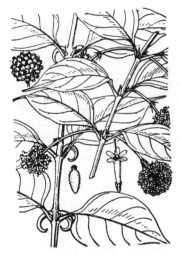

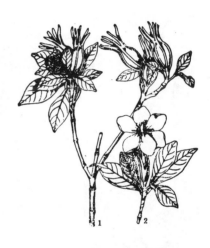

Gardenia jasminoides

Uncaria rhynchophylla

Gardenia
(Cape Jasmine)

Botanical name: *Gardenia jasminoides* (Rubiaceae)

Pharmaceutical name: Fructus Gardeniae

Chinese name: *chien-chih, chih-tzu* 梔子

Constituents: gardenin, crocin, chlorogenin, tannin, mannitol

Properties and actions: cold; bitter. Antipyretic, hemostatic, antiphlogistic.

Indications: anxiety, insomnia, jaundice, thirst, fever, ophthalmia, hemoptysis, hemorrhage, dysentery, diarrhea, melena, hematuria, intoxication, ulcers, styes, canker sores, toothache, mastitis, snake bite

Gastrodia

Botanical name: *Gastrodia elata* (Orchidaceae)

Pharmaceutical name: Rhizoma Gastrodiae

Chinese name: *tien-ma* 天麻

From *Shen Nung's Herbal* (superior drug)

Properties and actions: neutral, biting to taste. Dispels flatus, quiets spasms.

Indications: headache, vertigo, epilepsy, monoplegia, spasms in the arms and legs, pain in the waist and knees

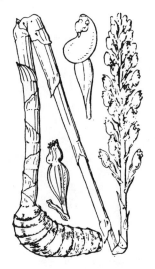

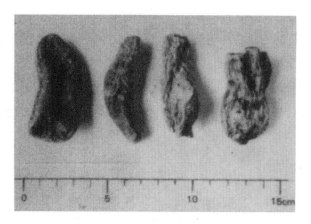

Rhizoma Gastrodiae

Gastrodia elata

Gelatin

Pharmaceutical name: Gelatinum Asini—gelatinous lump of asshide

Chinese name: *a-chiao* 阿膠

Constituents: proteamino acid, glutin

Actions: treats yin weakness

Indications: insomnia, phthisis, cough, anthrax with suppuration, hematemesis, hemoptysis, rectal bleeding, difficult urination

Gentian (Chin-chiu)

Botanical name: *Gentiana macrophylla* (Gentianaceae)

Pharmaceutical name: Radix Gentianae Macrophyllae

Chinese name: *chin-chiu* 秦艽

From *Shen Nung's Herbal*

Properties and actions: bland, bitter, and pungent. Promotes diuresis and sweating, cools, relieves pain.

Indications: rheumatism, dysuria, diarrhea, fever, bonesteaming fever, children's hernia fever, tidal fever, carbuncles, jaundice, paralysis, pain, spasms, intestinal bleeding

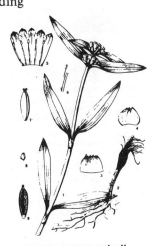

Gentiana macrophylla

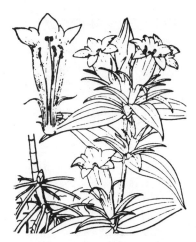

Gentiana scabra var. *buergeri*

Gentian

Botanical name: *Gentiana scabra* (Gentianaceae)

Pharmaceutical name: Radix Gentianae

Chinese name: *lung-tan* 龍膽

From *Shen Nung's Herbal* (general drug)

Constituents: bitter glycosides gentiopicrin, gentiamarin, gentiin; the trisaccharide gentianose

Properties and actions: cold, bitter and biting to taste. Stomachic, carminative, and purgative agent.

Indications: chills, fever, agitated epilepsy, intercostal pain, ophthalmia, sore throat, bitter taste in the mouth, swelling carbuncles

Ginger

Botanical name: *Zingiber officinale* (Zingiberaceae)

Pharmaceutical name: Rhizoma Zingiberis

Chinese name: *chiang, sheng-chiang* 薑，生薑

Constituents: essential oils, fat, gingerol, resin, zingerone, phellandrene, camphene, cineol, borneol, citral, gingerol

Properties and actions: warm; acrid. Sialogogue, sternatory, rubefacient, stimulant, carminative.

Indications: colds, sputum, nausea, asthma, distention, food poisoning, yang deficiencies, slow pulse, cold extremities

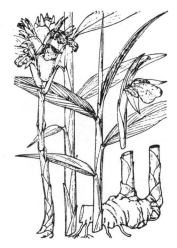

Zingiber officinale

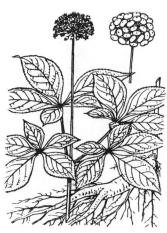

Panax ginseng

Ginseng

Botanical name: *Panax ginseng, P. quinquefolium* (Araliaceae)

Pharmaceutical name: Radix Ginseng

Chinese name: *jen-shen, hsi-yang-shen* 人參，西洋參

Constituents: glycoside panaquilon, saporin panaxin, phytosterols, vitamins B_1 and B_2; a hormone, resin, mucilage, starch

Properties and actions: cold; bitter with mildly sweet taste. Tonic. Promotes mental stability, dispels "fire," promotes production of body fluids.

Indications: weakness, nausea, diarrhea, sweating, cough, asthma, convulsions, pulmonary atrophy, weak fever, impaired memory, thirst, "stomach fire"—all conformations stemming from lack of blood or body fluids

Gleditsia
(Chinese Locust or Soap Bean Tree)

Botanical name: *Gleditsia sinensis* (Leguminosae)

Pharmaceutical name: Fructus Gleditsiae—dried pods

Chinese name: *tsao-chiao* 皂角

From *Shen Nung's Herbal*

Constituents: saponins

Properties and actions: warm; pungent and salty. Stimulant and expectorant. Relieves constipation, resolves phlegm, loosens congestion.

Indications: apoplexy, epilepsy, asthma with expectoration, constipation

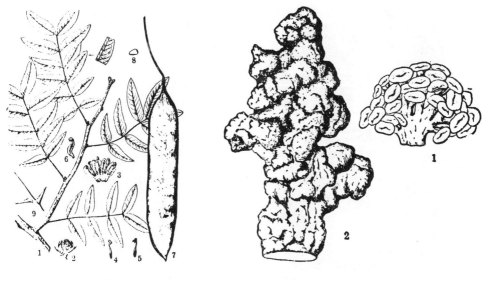

Gleditsia sinensis　　　　　　　　　　*Grifola umbellata*

Grifolia (Polyporus)
(Chuling)

Botanical name: *Grifolia umbellata* (*Polyporus umbellatus*) (Basidiomycetes)

Pharmaceutical name: Sclerotium Polypori—entire fungus is used

Chinese name: *chu-ling* 豬苓

Properties and actions: diuretic

Indications: dysuria, edema, abdominal distention, leukorrhea, gonorrheal discharge

Gypsum

Chinese name: *shih-kao* 石膏

Constituents: calcium sulphate, ferrous sulphate, magnesium sulphate, aluminum hydroxide

Properties and actions: very cold; biting, yet pleasant to taste. Relieves heat, improves muscle function, treats abscesses and ulcers.

Indications: moderate fever, extreme thirst, dry mouth and tongue, perspiration, speech disorders, mental illness, rapid pulse, rashes, cough, asthma, sunstroke, headache, toothache and inflamed gums

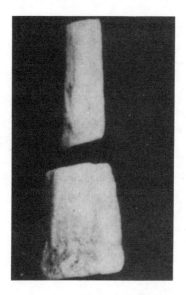

Gypsum

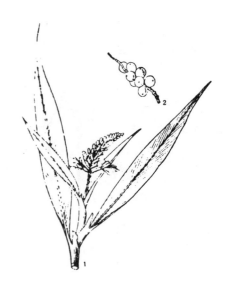

Alpinia oxyphylla

Ichihjen (Black Cardamon)

Botanical name: *Alpinia oxyphylla* (Zingiberaceae)

Pharmaceutical name: Fructus Alpiniae

Chinese name: *i-chih-jen* 益智仁

Properties and actions: warm; pungent. A stomachic, stimulant, astringent, tonic.

Indications: chilling, abdominal pain, spermatorrhea, nocturnal polyuria

Inula
(Elecampane)

Botanical name: *Inula britannica* var. *chinensis* (Compositae)

Pharmaceutical name: Flos Inulae

Chinese name: *hsuan-fu-hua* 旋覆花

From *Shen Nung's Herbal*

Constituents: inulin, flavone

Properties and actions: warm; salty. A mild poison. Expectorant, stomachic, tonic, alterative, deobstruent, carminative, laxative. Warms, resolves phlegm, promotes fluid elimination.

Indications: cough, asthma, intestinal fullness, pain in the hypochondria, pulmonary disorders, edema of the abdomen

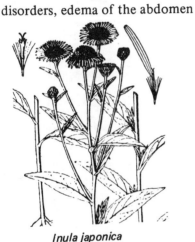

Inula japonica

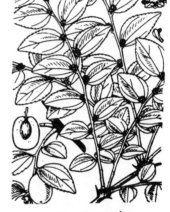

Zizyphus sativa

Jujube
(Chinese Date or Zizyphus)

Botanical name: *Zizyphus sativa, Z. inermis* (Rhamnaceae)

Pharmaceutical name: Fructus Zizyphi Sativae

Chinese name: *hung-tsao, ta-tsao* 大棗

Constituents: mucilage, sugar, protein, fat, tannin, betulin, betulinic acid, stearic acid, palmitic acid, linolenic acid

Properties and actions: neutral; sour to taste. Regulates cardiac and pulmonary functions, treats weak stomach and spleen, calms nerves.

Indications: lack of vigor, insufficient blood and body fluids, insomnia, dizziness, clamminess, forgetfulness

Juncus
(Rush or Bulrush)

Botanical name: *Juncus decipiens* (Juncaceae)

Pharmaceutical name: Medulla Juncus—dried pith

Chinese name: *teng-hsin-tsao* 燈心草

From *Kai pao pen tsao*

Constituents: arabinose, xylan

Properties and actions: cool. Sedative, diuretic.

Indications: gonorrhea, dysuria, insomnia from stress

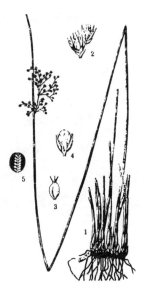

Juncus decipiens

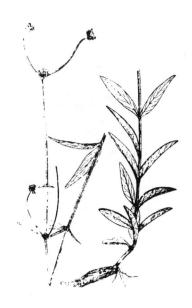

Knoxia valerianoides

Knoxia

Botanical name: *Knoxia valerianoides* (Rubiaceae)

Pharmaceutical name: Radix Knoxiae

Chinese name: *ta-chi* 大戟

Properties and actions: cool; bitter, pungent, sweet. It is thought to be poisonous and scratches the throat. Dispels water, sputum, and saliva; eliminates edema.

Indications: pain in the chest and back, dry heaves, *ku* disease, dropsy, persistent nausea and vomiting, diarrhea

Lard

Pharmaceutical name: Oleum Sus—accumulated fat in the abdomen and around the
kidneys of a pig

Chinese name: *tun-chih* 豚脂

Constituents: oleine, starine

Properties and actions: lubricant. Used as a base for ointments.

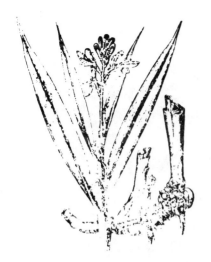

Alpinia officinarum

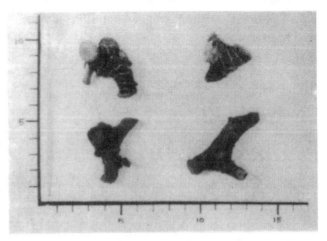

Rhizoma Alpiniae

Lesser Galangal

Botanical name: *Alpinia officinarum* (Zingiberaceae)

Pharmaceutical name: Rhizoma Alpiniae

Chinese name: *kao-liang-chiang, liang-chiang* 良薑

Constituents: essential oils (galangol, cineol, eugenol, pinene, cardinene, methyl
cinnamate), sesquiterpene, dioxyflavonol

Properties and actions: anodyne, stomachic

Indications: chills, abdominal pain, cold spleen, vomiting, diarrhea, nausea, malaria
with chills

213

Licorice

Botanical name: *Glycyrrhiza uralensis, G. glabra* (Leguminosae)

Pharmaceutical name: Radix Glycyrrhizae

Chinese name: *tiao-tsao, kan-ts'ao* 甘草

Constituents: glycyrrhizin, glucose, protein, mannite, asparagin, resin, calcium, manganese, ammonium, urease, glucuronic acid, saccharase

Properties and actions: neutral; pleasant to taste. Relaxant. Relieves intoxication, loosens phlegm, supplements energy.

Indications: spleen weakness, fatigue, fever, stomachache, thirst, cough, palpitations, throat pain and swelling, vomiting, diarrhea

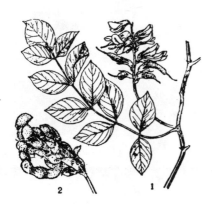

Glycyrrhiza uralensis

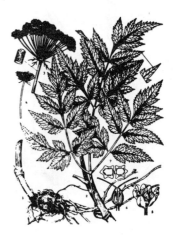

Ligusticum sinense

Ligusticum (Kao-pen)
(Wax Tree)

Botanical name: *Ligusticum sinense* (Umbelliferae)

Pharmaceutical name: Radix Ligustici Sinensis

Chinese name: *kao-pen* 藁本

From *Shen Nung's Herbal*

Constituents: syringin, invertin

Properties and actions: warm; bitter, pungent. Stimulant, antispasmodic, antiarthritic, deobstruent, nutrient tonic. Dispels "wind," chills, moisture, and toxin. Added to cosmetic preparations because of its benefits to the skin and its fragrance.

Indications: headache, women's hernia, cramping pain in the abdomen, *acne rosacea*

Lindera

Botanical name: *Lindera strychnifolia* (Lauraceae)

Pharmaceutical name: Radix Linderae

Chinese name: *wu-yao* 烏藥

From *Kai pao pen tsao* (973 A.D.)

Constituents: linderane, linderene, linderene acetate

Properties and actions: warm-natured; slightly biting to taste. Expels gas and disperses cold, corrects energy and relieves congestion, reduces inflammation and alleviates pain.

Indications: pain and distention in the chest, nausea and vomiting, frequent micturition, hernia

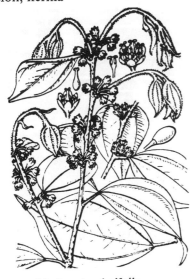

Lindera strychnifolia

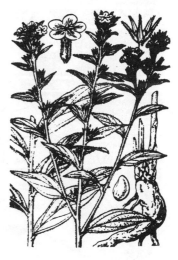

Lithospermum erythrorhizon

Lithospermum
(Groomwell, Red-Rooted)

Botanical name: *Lithospermum erythrorhizon, L. officinale* (Boraginaceae)

Pharmaceutical name: Radix Lithospermi

Chinese name: *tzu-ts'ao* 紫草

Constituents: the two crystalline coloring matters shikonin and acetyl-shikonin

Properties and actions: cold; pleasant, yet biting. Clears fevers, cools blood, detoxifies and lubricates the intestines.

Indications: burns, cuts, scalds, bleeding, oozing dermatitis, abscesses, constipation

Longan

Botanical name: *Euphoria longana* (Sapindaceae)
Pharmaceutical name. Arillus Longanae—undried aril of the evergreen tree
Chinese name: *lung-yen-jou* 龍眼肉
From *Shen Nung's Herbal* (superior drug)
Constituents: glucose, sucrose, tartaric acid, vitamins A and B
Properties and actions: nutritive, tonic, hematinic
Indications: amnesia, palpitations caused by fear, insomnia

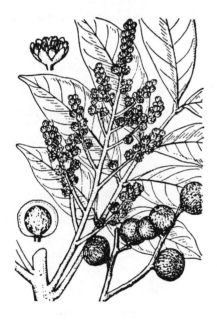

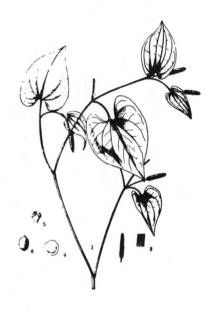

Euphoria longana   *Piper longum*

Long Pepper (Piper)

Botanical name: *Piper longum* (Piperaceae)
Pharmaceutical name: Fructus Piperis Longi—unripe fruit spike
Chinese name: *pi-pa* 蓽茇
Constituents: volatile oil, the alkaloid piperine
Properties and actions: warm; pungent. Antipyretic, carminative.
Indications: chills, vomiting, gastric fullness and aching, watery diarrhea, headache, toothache, nasal suppuration

Lonicera

Botanical name: *Lonicera japonica* (Caprifoliaceae)

Pharmaceutical name: Flos Lonicerae

Chinese name: *chin-yin-hua* 金銀花

From *Pen tsao kang mu*

Constituents: The stems contain saponin; the leaves, 8% tannin; the flowers, 1% inositol.

Properties and actions: cooling properties; pleasant yet bitter to taste. Clears fevers and detoxifies.

Indications: primary fever of the warm diseases, swelling carbuncles, scabies

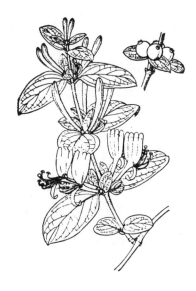

Lonicera japonica

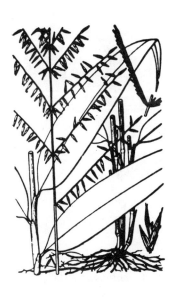

Lophatherum gracile

Lophatherum

Botanical name: *Lophatherum gracile* (Gramineae)

Pharmaceutical name: Herba Lophatheri

Chinese name: *tan-chu-yeh* 淡竹葉

Properties and actions: cold; slightly sweet. Clears fever, dispels feelings of agitation and apprehension, promotes diuresis.

Indications: irritability, red urine, oliguria

Loranthus

Botanical name: *Loranthus yakoriki, L. parasiticus* (Loranthaceae)

Pharmaceutical name: Ramulus Loranthi

Chinese name: *sang-chi-sheng* 桑寄生

From *Shen Nung's Herbal* (superior drug)

Constituents: caryophyllin, meso-inositol

Properties and actions: neutral, bitter to taste. Nourishes blood, moisturizes sinews, eliminates flatus, clears passageways.

Indications: backache, weakness of feet and knees, rheumatism, numbness and pain, stiff joints, puerperal difficulties, inadequate lactation

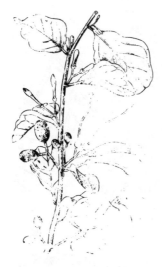

Loranthus parasiticus

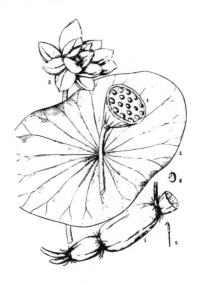

Nelumbo nucifera

Lotus

Botanical name: *Nelumbo nucifera* (Nymphaceae)

Pharmaceutical name: Fructus Nelumbonis

Chinese name: *shih-lien-tzu* 石蓮子

From *Shen Nung's Herbal*

Constituents: starch, vitamin C, asparagin, nelumbine

Properties and actions: cold; bitter. Tonic.

Indications: chronic dysentery, leukorrhea, gonorrhea, spermatorrhea, insomnia, neurasthenia

Lycium Bark
(Boxthorn or Chinese Wolfberry)

Botanical name: *Lycium chinense* (Solanaceae)

Pharmaceutical name: Cortex Radicis Lycii–dried root bark

Chinese name: *ti-ku-pi*　地骨皮

From *Shen Nung's Herbal*

Constituents: betaine, a polyterpene, physaline, vitamin A

Properties and actions: cool; bitter. Antitussive, antipyretic.

Indications: hemoptysis, cough, fever from stress, tuberculosis, diabetes

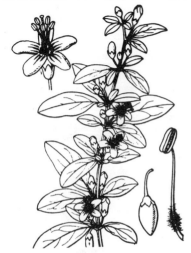

Lycium chinense

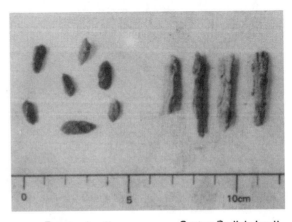

Fructus Lycii　　　　　Cortex Radicis Lycii

Lycium Fruit

Botanical name: *Lycium barbarum, Lycium chinense* (Solanaceae)

Pharmaceutical name: Fructus Lycii

Chinese name: *kou-chi-tzu*　枸杞子

From *Shen Nung's Herbal* (superior drug)

Constituents: betaine, a polyterpene, physaline, vitamin A

Properties and actions: Fruit has neutral properties, pleasant to taste. Strengthens the kidneys and restores semen, nourishes the liver and clears vision. Root bark has "*han*" (chill) properties, bitter to taste. Cools the blood and purges fire, clears pulmonary "heat."

Indications: weakness of the liver and kidneys, aching in the waist and knees, vertigo

Magnesium Sulphate (Mirabilitum)

Pharmaceutical name: Magnesii Sulfuricum

Chinese name: *mang-hsiao* 芒硝

Constituents: potassium nitrate, sodium nitrate, sodium chloride

Properties and actions: Laxative, expectorant. Reduces fever.

Indications: strong fever, constipation, sputum

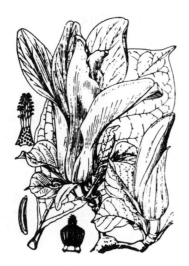

Magnolia liliflora

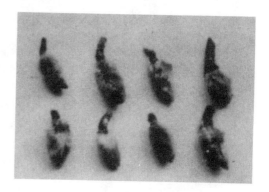

Flos Magnoliae Liliflorae

Magnolia Flower

Botanical name: *Magnolia liliflora, M. denudata, M. fargesii, M. salicifolia* (Magnoliaceae)

Pharmaceutical name: Flos Magnoliae Liliflorae

Chinese name: *hsin-i, mu-pi* 辛夷，木筆

Constituents: citral-eugenol, cineol, chavicol, methyl-ether, pinene, capric acid, oleic acid

Properties and actions: warm; acrid. Disperses heat, alleviates pain.

Indications: hot face and head, headache, stuffy nose

Magnolia Bark

Botanical name: *Magnolia officinalis, M. obovata* (Magnoliaceae)

Pharmaceutical name: Cortex Magnoliae

Chinese name: *ch'uan-hou-p'o* 川厚朴

Constituents: machilol, magnonal, magnocurarine, no-curare

Properties and actions: warm; bitter, acrid. Antispasmodic, stomachic, antiseptic.

Indications: gastritis, abdominal distention, nausea, cough, asthma, diarrhea

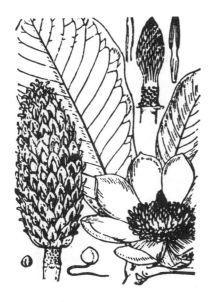

Magnolia obovata

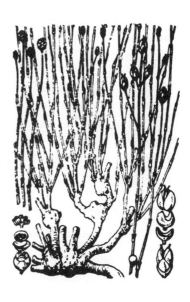

Ephedra sinica

Mahuang
(Ephedra)

Botanical name: *Ephedra sinica* (Ephedraceae)

Pharmaceutical name: Herba Ephedrae

Chinese name: *ma-huang* 麻黄

Constituents: ephedrine

Properties and actions: warm; acrid to taste. Bronchial dilator, diaphoretic. Stimulates respiration and heart beat, raises blood pressure.

Indications: asthma, typhus, fever, chills, bone and joint pain, cough, bronchitis, edema

221

Maltose

Acts as a nutrient, base, and dietary supplement.

Mint (Mentha)
(Field Mint, Pennyroyal)

Botanical name: *Mentha arvensis* var. *piperascens* (Labiatae)

Pharmaceutical name: Herba Menthae

Chinese name: *po-ho* 薄荷

Constituents: menthol, menthone, *d*-piperitone, limonene, hexenolphenylacetate, ethylamylcarbinol, neomenthol

Properties and actions: cool, acrid, aromatic. Stomachic, carminative, stimulant, diaphoretic.

Indications: fever, headache, eye problems, sore throat, cough with expectoration, mouth abscess, toothache, itching, scrofula, scabies

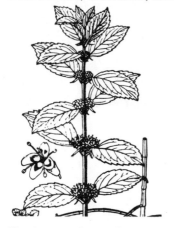

Mentha arvensis var. *piperascens*

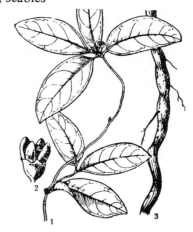

Morinda officinalis

Morinda

Botanical name: *Morinda officinalis* (Rubiaceae)

Pharmaceutical name: Radix Morindae

Chinese name: *pa-chi-tien* 巴戟天

From *Shen Nung's Herbal*

Properties and actions: mild and warm; pungent taste. Prevents loss of semen in nocturnal emissions, strengthens bones and sinews, eliminates rheumatism.

Morning Glory (Pharbitis)

Botanical name: *Pharbitis nil* (Convolvulaceae)
Pharmaceutical name: Semen Pharbitidis
Chinese name: *chien-niu-tzu* 牽牛子
From *Ming-i-pieh-lu*
Constituents: pharbitin
Properties and actions: hot; pungent. Poisonous. Diuretic, anthelmintic, deobstruent. Promotes menstruation, induces abortion.
Indications: edema, distention, sputum, beriberi, constipation, worms

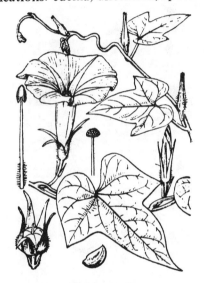

Pharbitis nil

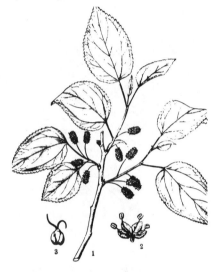

Morus alba

Morus
(Mulberry)

Botanical name: *Morus alba* (Moraceae)
Pharmaceutical name: Cortex Mori Albae
Chinese name: *sang-pai-pi* 桑白皮
From *Shen Nung's Herbal* (general drug)
Constituents: α, β-amyrin, sitosterol, resinotannol palmitic acid
Properties and actions: cold, acrid, yet pleasant to taste. Relieves lung congestion and promotes diuresis.
Indications: asthma, cough, internal heat in the lungs, hemoptysis, edema, abdominal distension

Moutan
(Tree Peony)

Botanical name: *Paeonia suffruticosa* (Ranunculaceae)
Pharmaceutical name: Cortex Moutan
Chinese name: *mou-tan-p'i* 牡丹皮
Constituents: ketone paeonol, glycosides, benzoic acid
Properties and actions: slightly chilling; biting and bitter. Antipyretic, emmenagogue.
Indications: amenorrhea, hemoptysis, blood disorders, ulcers, boils, abscesses, bruises, typhoid fever

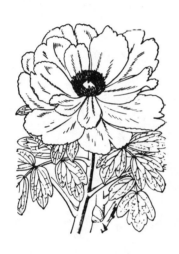

Paeonia suffruticosa

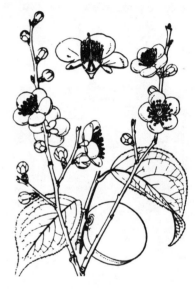

Prunus mume

Mume
(Dark Plum)

Botanical name: *Prunus mume* (Rosaceae)
Pharmaceutical name: Fructus Mume—fried half-ripe fruit
Chinese name: *wu-mei* 烏梅
From *Shen Nung's Herbal*
Constituents: hydrocyanic acid
Properties and actions: warm; sour, astringent. Carminative, antifebrile, antispasmodic.
Indications: persistent coughs, diarrhea, melena, intestinal worms, pyrosis, vomiting, thirst

Musk Deer

Scientific name: *Moschus moschiferus* (Cervidae)

Pharmaceutical name: Secretio Moschi. Dried secretion from preputial follicles.

Chinese name: *she-hsiang* 麝香

From *Shen Nung's Herbal*

Constituents: muskone

Properties: malodorous. Antispasmodic, cardiotonic, stimulant, analgesic.

Indications: fear-induced convulsions, apoplexy, coma, injuries resulting from falls, swelling carbuncles

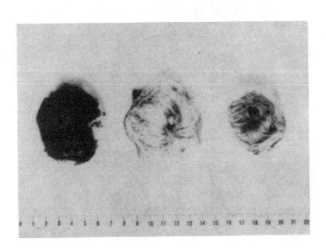

Secretio Moschi

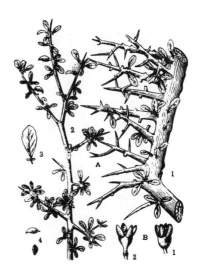

Commiphora myrrha

Myrrh

Botanical name: *Commiphora myrrha* (Burseraceae)

Pharmaceutical name: Myrrha

Chinese name: *mo-yao* 没藥

From *Kai pao pen tsao*

Constituents: resin, gum, essential oils

Properties and actions: antiseptic, hematonic, analgesic. Minimizes secretions.

Indications: swollen, painful carbuncles; injuries; stagnant blood; amenorrhea; pain in the chest and abdomen. Externally applied to scabies.

Nuphar

Botanical name: *Nuphar japonicum* (Nymphaeaceae)
Pharmaceutical name: Rhizoma Nuphario
Chinese name: *chuan-ku* 川骨
Constituents: nupharin, rhamnosan
Properties and actions: tonic
Indications: anemia, chills, irregular menstruation, gynecological conditions

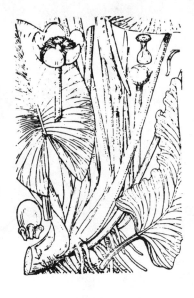

Nuphar japonicum

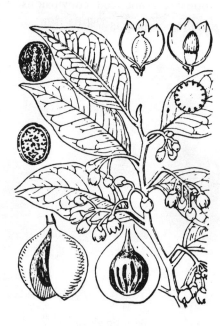

Myristica fragrans

Nutmeg

Botanical name: *Myristica fragrans* (Myristicaceae)
Pharmaceutical name: Semen Myristicae
Chinese name: *jou-tou-kou* 肉豆蔻
Constituents: volatile oil comprising *d*-camphene, *d*-pinene, dipentene, *d*-linalol, safrole, eugenol, iso-eugenol, *d*-borneol, *l*-terpineol, geraniol, myristicin
Properties and actions: warm; pungent. Carminative, stomachic. Warms, astringes.
Indications: diarrhea due to weakness and chills, chilling pain in the stomach, vomiting, food stagnancy, vomiting milk

226

Oakgall

Botanical name: *Galla halepensis*

Pharmaceutical name: dried gall from *Quercus infectoria* Olivier (oak tree) of the Fagaceae family. Caused by the parasite *Cynips gallae-tinctoriae* Olivier and gathered before the insects fly away.

Chinese name: *mo-shih-tzu* 没食子

Properties and actions: warm; slightly bitter and astringent. Nutgall is the chief source of tannic acid which has astringent and styptic properties and is an antidote for alkaloid poisoning.

Indications: persistent bloody diarrhea, spermatorrhea, night sweats. In powdered form, externally applied to stop yin sweating and bleeding from cuts.

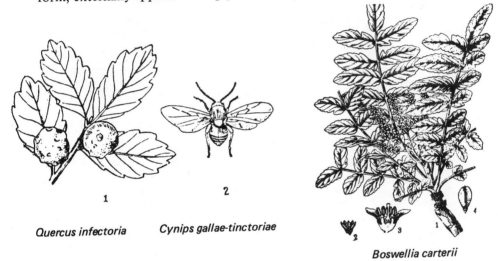

1
Quercus infectoria

2
Cynips gallae-tinctoriae

Boswellia carterii

Olibanum (Mastic)

Botanical name: *Boswellia carterii, B. neglecta* (Burseraceae)

Pharmaceutical name: Olibanum—dried mastic

Chinese name: *ju-hsiang* 乳香

From *Ming i pieh* lu (superior drug)

Constituents: resin, gum, essential oil, anisaldehyde, methylchavicol, enzymes, arabinose, dioxybenzene, xylose

Properties and actions: warm; bitter and acrid. Analgesic, astringent, sedative. Stimulates circulation, resolves bruises and clots, relieves pain.

Indications: carbuncles, cardiac and abdominal pain, wounds and injuries

Ophiopogon
(Lilyturf)

Botanical name: *Ophiopogon japonicus* (Liliaceae)
Pharmaceutical name: Radix Ophiopogonis
Chinese name: *mai-men-tung* 麥門冬
Constituents: mucilage, β-sitosterol, stigmasterol, vitamin A, ruscogenin
Properties and actions: slightly cold; pleasant yet bitter to taste. Antitussive, expectorant, emollient. Regulates lungs and heart.
Indications: weakness, cough, spitting blood, thirst, laryngitis

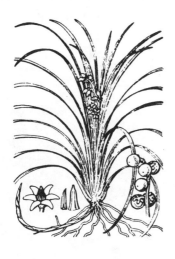

Ophiopogon japonicus

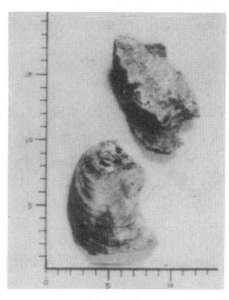

Concha Ostreae

Oyster Shell

Pharmaceutical name: Concha Ostreae
Chinese name: *mu-li* 牡蠣
Constituents: calcium carbonate, calcium phosphate
Properties and actions: slightly cool; salty and acrid. Antipyretic, antisudorific, expectorant. Moderates yang, stabilizes, clears fever, breaks up congestion.
Indications: yin weakness, inside heat, night sweats, nocturnal emissions, scrofula, malaria

Peony

Botanical name: *Paeonia lactiflora, P. albiflora, P. obovata* (Ranunculaceae)

Pharmaceutical name: Radix Paeoniae

Chinese name: *chih-shao, pai-shao* 赤芍，白芍

Constituents: paeoniflorin, asparagin, benzoic acid

Properties and actions: slightly cold; bitter and biting. Strengthens blood, regulates the liver, lessens perspiration, purifies yin.

Indications: chest pain, stomachache, dysentery, abdominal pain, anemia, sweating, night sweats, spasms of the arms and legs, menstrual irregularities, fever; yin weak conformation

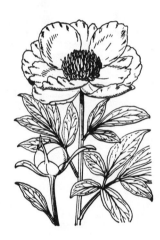

Paeonia lactiflora

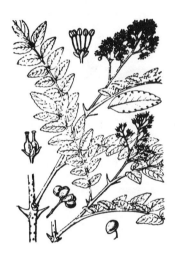

Zanthoxylum piperitum

Pepper

Botanical name: *Zanthoxylum piperitum, Z. bungei, Z. schinifolium, Z. simulans* (Rutaceae)

Pharmaceutical name: Fructus Zanthoxyli

Chinese name: *hua-chiao* 花椒

From *Shen Nung's Herbal* (inferior drug)

Constituents: essential oils

Properties and actions: warm; pungent. Vermifuge, aromatic, stomachic. Expels worms and parasites.

Indications: chills and pain in the abdomen, vomiting, watery diarrhea

Perilla

Botanical name: *Perilla frutescens* var. *crispa, P. ocymoides* (Labiatae)

Pharmaceutical name: Folium Perillae

Chinese name: *tzu-su, pai-tzu-su* 紫蘇，白紫蘇

Constituents: essential oil perilla, aldehyde, *d*-pinene, *l*-limonene, perillanine

Properties and actions: warm; acrid, aromatic. Antitussive, stomachic, antiseptic. Dispels cold, corrects *ch'i* imbalance, relieves asthma, quiets fetus, detoxifies.

Indications: cough, asthma, abdominal and cardiac distention, seafood poisoning

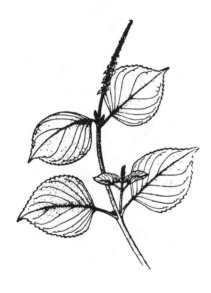

Perilla frutescens

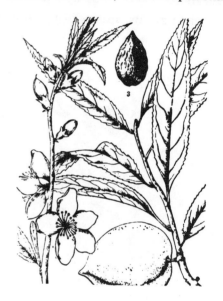

Prunus persica

Persica
(Peach)

Botanical name: *Prunus persica* (Rosaceae)

Pharmaceutical name: Semen Persicae

Chinese name: *pi-tao-kan, t'ao-jen* 桃仁

Constituents: volatile oil, amygdalin, emulsin

Properties and actions: antitussive, sedative

Indications: congested blood, mental instability, injuries from falling, constipation amenorrhea

Phellodendron Tree
(Cork Tree)

Botanical name: *Phellodendron chinense, P. amurense, P. wilsonii* (Rutaceae)

Pharmaceutical name: Cortex Phellodendri

Chinese name: *huang-po* 黃柏

Constituents: alkaloids berberine, palmatine; mucilage; limonine

Properties and actions: cold; bitter. Expectorant, stomachic, cathartic.

Indications: sputum, chest distress, impaired digestion, abdominal distention, constipation, hemorrhoids, bloody stools, aching bones, canker sores, lameness, paralysis, conjunctivitis, tinnitus, boils, gonorrhea, leukorrhea, bloody vaginal discharge

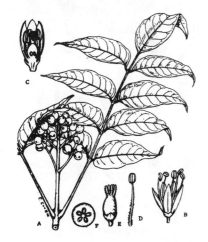

Phellodendron wilsonii

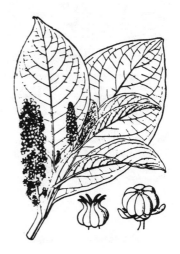

Phytolacca esculenta

Phytolacca
(Poke Root)

Botanical name: *Phytolacca esculenta* (Phytolaccaceae)

Pharmaceutical name: Radix Phytolaccae

Chinese name: *shang-lu* 商陸

From Shen Nung's Nerbal

Constituents: saponin, formic acid, tannin, phytolacein, fatty oil, resin, sugar

Properties and actions: cool; bitter. Poisonous. Discharges stagnant water.

Indications: edema, distention, fullness. Externally used for foul sores.

Picrasma

Botanical name: *Picrasma ailanthoides* (Simarubaceae)

Pharmaceutical name: Lignum Picrasmae. The drug is derived from the center of the trunk of the tree.

Chinese name: *ku-mu* 苦木

Properties and actions: bitter. Stomachic.

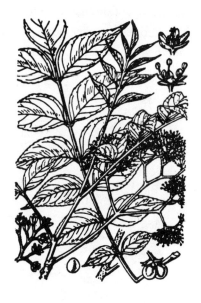

Picrasma ailanthoides

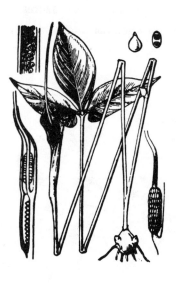

Pinellia ternata

Pinellia

Botanical name: *Pinellia ternata* (Araceae)

Pharmaceutical name: Rhizoma Pinelliae

Chinese name: *pan-hsia, su-hsia* 半夏

Constituents: β-sitosterol, *d*-glucoside, choline, an amino acid, homogentisic acid, fat, ash

Properties and actions: warm; acrid. Toxic. Reduces expectoration, subdues nausea, strengthens spleen, stops bleeding, resolves phlegm, reduces inflammation.

Indications: cough, vomiting, asthma, chest distress, cerebral hemorrhage, vertigo, headache, insomnia, painful swelling

Plantago
(Plantain)

Botanical name: *Plantago asiatica* (Plantaginaceae)
Pharmaceutical name: *Semen Plantaginis*
Chinese name: *che-chien-tzu* 車前子
From *Shen Nung's Herbal* (superior drug)

Constituents: plantenolic acid, succinic acid

Properties and actions: cool; sweet. Diuretic, antitussive, antipurgative. Clears fevers, detoxifies.

Indications: diarrhea with fever, gonorrhea, hematuria, carbuncles, moist spasms, ophthalmia with swelling and pain

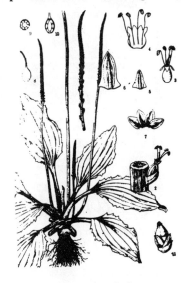

Plantago asiatica

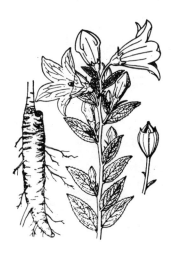

Platycodon grandiflorum

Platycodon
(Balloon Flower, Broad Bluebell)

Botanical name: *Platycodon grandiflorum, P. glaucum* (Campanulaceae)
Pharmaceutical name: Radix Platycodi
Chinese name: *chieh-keng* 桔梗
Constituents: saponins, inulin, platycodigenin, stigmasterol, *d*-spinasterol, phytosterol
Properties and actions: expectorant. Reduces swelling, promotes pus drainage.
Indications: cough, sore throat, expectoration of blood and pus

Polygala
(Chinese Seneca or Milkwort)

Botanical name: *Polygala senega, P. tenuifolia, P. sibirica* (Polygalaceae)

Pharmaceutical name: Radix Polygalae

Chinese name: *yuan-chih* 遠志

Constituents: tannin, anthraquinone derivatives, an essential oil, a volatile alkaloid, avicularin, quercite, rutin

Properties and actions: warm; acrid, pleasant to taste. Expectorant, sedative. Reduces swelling.

Indications: melancholia, impaired memory, palpitation, cough, excessive sputum

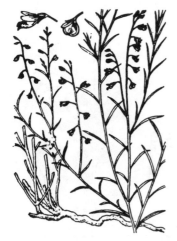

Polygala tenuifolia

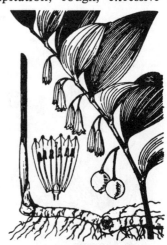

Polygonatum officinale

Polygonatum
(Solomon's Seal)

Botanical name: *Polygonatum officinale* (Liliaceae)

Pharmaceutical name: Rhizoma Polygonati Officinalis

Chinese name: *yu-chu* 玉竹

Constituents: glycosides convallarin and convallamarin, mucilage

Properties and actions: slightly cold; sweet. Tonic, antiarthritic, demulcent. Stimulates appetite, increases peristalsis, slows the heart, raises arterial tension, slows and deepens respiration, cools, sedates.

Indications: fever, thirst, rheumatism, cough, spontaneous sweating, fever due to weakness and fatigue

Polygonatum
(Solomon's Seal)

Botanical name: *Polygonatum sibiricum, P. multiflorum* var. *longifolium* (Liliaceae)

Pharmaceutical name: Rhizoma Polygonati

Chinese name: *huang-ching* 黃精

From *Ming-i-pieh-lu*

Constituents: starch, fat, ash

Properties and actions: bland; sweet. Tonic, antiarthritic, demulcent, lenitive, prophylactic. Treats weakness of spleen, stomach, and lungs.

Indications: cough, thirst

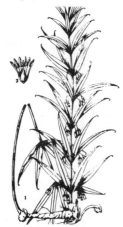

Polygonatum sibiricum

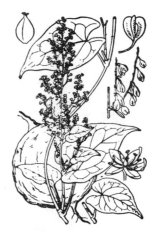

Polygonum multiflorum

Polygonum (Ho-shou-wu)
(Chinese Cornbind)

Botanical name: *Polygonum multiflorum* (Polygonaceae)

Pharmaceutical name: Radix Polygoni Multiflori. Commonly sold in flat, oblong, or round pieces.·

Chinese name: *ho-shou-wu* 何首烏

Constituents: starch, lecithin, chrysophanol

Properties and actions: warm; bitter and sweet taste. Astringent. Nourishes the liver and kidneys, promotes fertility, strengthens sinews and bones, builds vitality.

Indications: emissions, leukorrhea, lower back pain, knee pain, anal fistula, tumors, piles, postpartum and menstrual difficulties, colds, diarrhea

Conformation: yin weak

Poria (Hoelen)
(China Root)

Botanical name: *Poria cocos* (Basidiomycetes)
Pharmaceutical name: Sclerotium Poriae—the fungus growing around pine roots
Chinese name: *fu-ling, fu-shen* 茯苓，茯神
Constituents: pectin, albuminoid, pachymose, ergoseerol, eburicoic acid, pacymic acid
Properties and actions: neutral; pleasant taste. Diuretic, sedative. Treats spleen and stomach.
Indications: cardiac disease, impaired memory, swelling, intestinal and vesicle heat, brownish urine, sputum, diarrhea, difficult urination, anxiety, insomnia

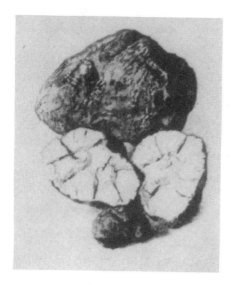

Poria cocos

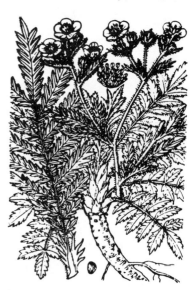

Potentilla chinensis

Potentilla
(Chinese Silver Weed)

Botanical name: *Potentilla chinensis* (Rosaceae)
Pharmaceutical name: Radix Potentillae Chinensis
Chinese name: *wei-ling-ts'ai* 委陵菜
From *Shen Nung's Herbal*
Properties and actions: cool; bitter. Eliminates fever, cools the blood.
Indications: fever toxin, bloody diarrhea, nosebleeds, warm malaria

Prunella
(Selfheal or Heal-all)

Botanical name: *Prunella vulgaris* (Labiatae)
Pharmaceutical name: Spica Prunellae
Chinese name: *hsia-ku-tsao* 夏枯草
From *Shen Nung's Herbal*
Constituents: an essential oil, a bitter principle
Properties and actions: warm; bitter and pungent. Antirheumatic, alterative, tonic.
Indications: scrofula; red, swelling, aching eyes; photophobia; tearing; fever; leukorrhea

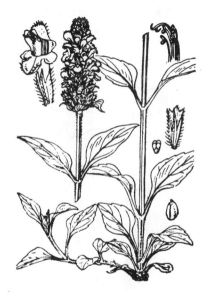

Prunella vulgaris

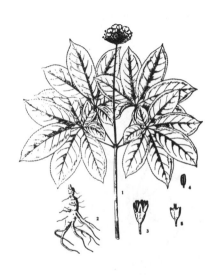

Panax pseudoginseng

Pseudoginseng

Botanical name: *Panax pseudoginseng* (Araliaceae)
Pharmaceutical name: Radix Pseudoginseng
Chinese name: *san-chi* 三七
Properties and actions: warm; sweet and slightly bitter. Hemostatic, discutient, analgesic. Dispels stagnancy. Can be used internally or externally.
Indications: hemoptysis, nosebleeds, metrorrhagia, unceasing lochia after childbirth, carbuncles, contusions

Psoralea
(Scurfy Pea)

Botanical name: *Psoralea corylifolia* (Leguminosae)
Pharmaceutical name: Semen Psoraleae
Chinese name: *pu-ku-chih* 補骨脂
Constituents: fatty oil, an alkaloid, psoralein or paraline
Properties and actions: very warm; pungent and bitter. Aphrodisiac, genital tonic. Tones the kidneys, promotes yang.
Indications: sexual incompetency, impotence, chilling and weakness of the spleen and kidneys, chilling pain in the lower back and knees, chilling diarrhea, enuresis, polyuria, urinary incontinence in children, discomforts of pregnancy, threatened abortion

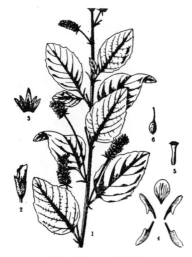

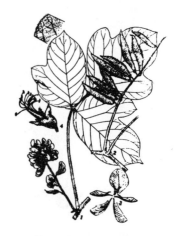

Psoralea corylifolia   *Pueraria pseudo-hirsuta*

Pueraria
(Kudzu Vine or Arrowroot Vine)

Botanical name: *Pueraria thunbergiana* (Leguminosae)
Pharmaceutical name: Radix Puerariae
Chinese name: *ko-ken* 葛根
Constituents: starch, saponin
Properties and actions: neutral; pleasant to taste. Antipyretic, refrigerant, stimulant.
Indications: fever, thirst, headache, stiff neck, diarrhea, dysentery, alcoholic intoxication

Quisqualis
(Rangoon Creeper)

Botanical name: *Quisqualis indica* (Combretaceae)
Pharmaceutical name: Fructus Quisqualis
Chinese name: *shih-chun-tzu* 使君子
From *Kai pao pen tsao*
Properties and actions: bland;sweet. Vermifugal. Eliminates malnutrition, kills parasites.
Indications: abdominal pain due to parasites, tabes mesentericus in children, sluggish peristalsis in infants

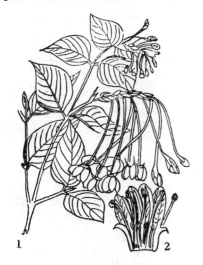

Quisqualis indica

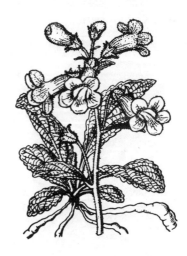

Rehmannia glutinosa

Rehmannia
(Chinese Foxglove)

Botanical name: *Rehmannia glutinosa* (Scrophulariaceae)
Pharmaceutical name: Radix Rehmanniae
Chinese name: *ti-huang, sheng-ti* 地黄
Constituents: glycosides, saponins, tannin, resins, β-sitosterol, vitamin A, mannitol
Properties and actions: the crude drug is cool, bitter, but pleasant to taste; processed it is warm. Cardiotonic, diuretic, hemostatic. Promotes salivation, nourishes yin, and supplements the blood.
Indications: thirst, fever, eruptions, hemoptysis, bleeding, deafness, vertigo, premature graying, difficult urination

Rhubarb

Botanical name: *Rheum palmatum, R. officinale, R. tanguticum* (Polygonaceae)
Pharmaceutical name: Rhizoma Rhei
Chinese name: *ta-huang* 大黃
Constituents: chryzophanic acid, chrysophanein, rhein, emodin, aloe emodin, rheochrysin, alizarin, glucogallin, tetrarin, catechin, anthraquinone derivatives, tannin, calcium oxalate
Properties and actions: cold; bitter. Stomachic, laxative.
Indications: fever, extravasated blood, constipation, speech disorders, mental instability, indigestion, chest distress, dysentery, stomachache, edema, amenorrhea, furunculosis, burns

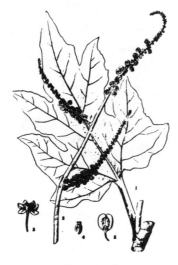

Rheum palmatum

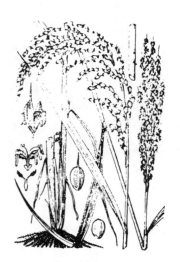

Oryza sativa

Rice (Oryza)

Botanical name: *Oryza sativa* (Gramineae)
Pharmaceutical name: Semen Oryzae
Chinese name: *hsien-mi, keng-mi* 秈米，粳米
Constituents: starch, protein, fat, amylase, vitamins A, B, C, D, and E
Properties and actions: stomachic, tonic. Stabilizes pulmonary and intestinal functions.
Indications: weak stomach and spleen, poor appetite, indigestion, distended chest and abdomen

Rosa
(Cherokee Rose)

Botanical name: *Rosa laevigata* (Rosaceae)

Pharmaceutical name: Fructus Rosae Laevigatae

Chinese name: *chin-ying-tzu* 金櫻子

From *Shu pen tsao*

Constituents: malic acid, citric acid, tannin, sugar, resin

Properties and actions: sour. Astringent and tonic. Detoxifies, stabilizes the kidneys, aids menstrual regularity.

Indications: nocturnal emissions, enuresis, frequent urination, prolonged diarrhea with a weak spleen

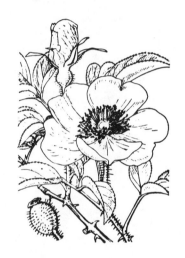

Rosa laevigata

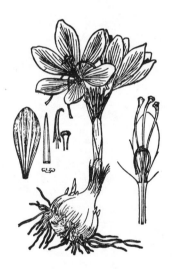

Crocus sativus

Saffron

Botanical name: *Crocus sativus* (Iridaceae)

Pharmaceutical name: Stigma Croci

Chinese name: *fan-hung-hua* 番紅花

Constituents: crocetin, pikrocrocin, crocin, essential oil, phosphatid, phytoseter-inester, pinene, terpene, cineol

Properties and actions: bland; sweet

Indications: menoxenia, prolonged menstruation, difficult labor, dead fetus, absence of lochia, contusions, pain caused by blood occlusion

Sandal Wood (Santalum)

Botanical name: *Santalum album* (Santalaceae)
Pharmaceutical name: Lignum Santali Albi
Chinese name: *tan-hsiang* 檀香
From *Ming i pieh lu*
Constituents: β-santalol, essential oils
Properties and actions: urinary antiseptic, analgesic
Indications: abdominal pain, vomiting, difficult breathing

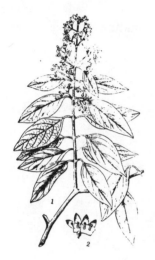

Santalum album

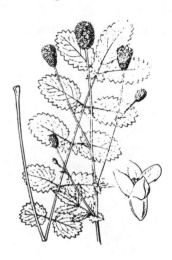

Sanguisorba officinalis

Sanguisorba
(Burnet)

Botanical name: *Sanguisorba officinalis* (Rosaceae)
Pharmaceutical name: Radix Sanguisorbae—dried roots
Chinese name: *ti-yu* 地榆
From *Shen Nung's Herbal*
Constituents: tannin, flavones, sanguisorbin
Properties and actions: slightly cool; bitter. Styptic, astringent, vulnerary, anodyne.
Indications: bloody diarrhea, anal fistula, metrorrhagia, postpartum difficulties, wounds, ulcers, dysentery, hemorrhages, snake and insect bites, skin diseases

242

Saussurea
(Costus)

Botanical name: *Saussurea lappa* (Compositae)

Pharmaceutical name: Radix Saussureae

Chinese name: *kuang-mu-hsiang* 廣木香

Constituents: the alkaloid saussurine, essential oils (costulactone, costol, costene, camphene, phellandrene)

Properties and actions: warm; biting, bitter. Stomachic. Promotes energy circulation.

Indications: indigestion, distended abdomen, abdominal pains, stomachache, vomiting, diarrhea, dysentery

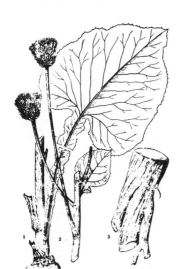

Saussurea lappa

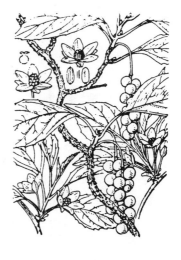

Schizandra chinensis

Schizandra

Botanical name: *Schizandra chinensis* (Schisandraceae)

Pharmaceutical name: Fructus Schizandrae

Chinese name: *pei-wu-wei* 北五味

Constituents: seed oil (schizandrin, schizandrol) and essential oil (ylangene)

Properties and actions: sour, aromatic. Strengthens lungs and kidneys, stimulates body fluids, stops perspiration.

Indications: cough, asthma, thirst, night sweats, nocturnal emissions

Schizonepeta
(Chinchieh)

Botanical name: *Schizonepeta tenuifolia* (Labiatae)
Pharmaceutical name: Herba Schizonepetae
Chinese name: *chin-chieh* 荆芥
Constituents: *d*-menthone, *d*-limonene
Properties and actions: antipyretic, hemostatic
Indications: colds, fever, chills, headache, sore throat, furunculosis, scabies, cerebra hemorrhage with aphasia, postnatal hemorrhage, hematemesis, hemoptysis rectal bleeding

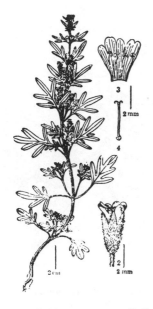

Schizonepeta tenuifolia

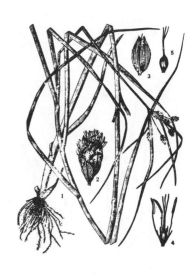

Scirpus yagara

Scirpus

Botanical name: *Scirpus yagara* (Cyperaceae)
Pharmaceutical name: Rhizoma Scirpi—dried rhizomes with cortex removed
Chinese name: *ching-san-leng* 荆三稜
Properties and actions: bland; bitter. Stomachic, tonic, deobstruent, wound healer. Stimulates menstrual flow, promotes milk production in nursing mothers.
Indications: dysmenorrhea, heart pain, abdominal pain, postpartum stagnancy

Scrophularia
(Ningpo Figwort)

Botanical name: *Scrophularia ningpoensis* (Scrophulariaceae)

Pharmaceutical name: Radix Scrophulariae

Chinese name: *hsuan-shen* 玄参

From *Shen Nung's Herbal*

Constituents: phytosterol, *l*-aspargine, harpagid

Properties and actions: slightly cold; bitter and salty. Anti-inflammative, antitoxic.
Nourishes yin, lowers heat, moisturizes heat dryness, promotes salivation.

Indications: sore throat, carbuncles, fever, thirst from stress

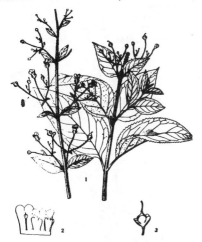

Scrophularia ningpoensis

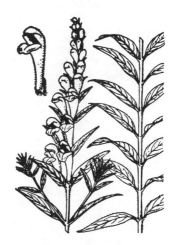

Scutellaria baicalensis

Scute
(Skullcap)

Botanical name: *Scutellaria baicalensis* (Labiatae)

Pharmaceutical name: Radix Scutellariae Baicalensis

Chinese name: *huang-ch'in* 黄芩

Constituents: essential oil, baicalin, flavone, baicalein, scutellarin, campesterol, stigmasterol

Properties and actions: cold; bitter. Reduces fever, removes moist heat, purges "fire," quiets the fetus.

Indications: congested lungs, cough, fever, thirst, dysentery, jaundice, sore eyes, furunculosis, hemoptysis

Sesame Oil

Botanical name: *Sesamum indicum* (Pedaliaceae)

Pharmaceutical name: Oleum Sesami

Chinese name: *hu-ma-you* 胡麻油

Constituents: sesamin, sesamol, oleic acid

Properties and actions: sedative, anti-inflammatory. Used as a base for ointments.

Indications: ringworm, itching, abscess, insect stings

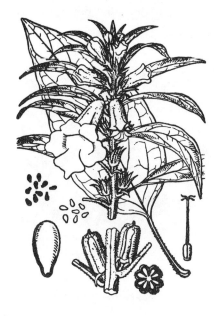

Sesamum indicum

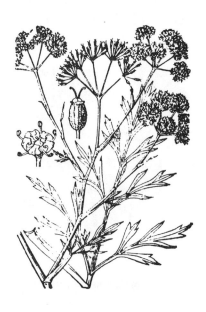

Siler divaricatum

Siler

Botanical name: *Ledebouriella seseloides, Ligusticum brachylobum, Siler divaricatum, Seseli delavayi* (Umbelliferae)

Pharmaceutical name: Rhizoma Seseli

Chinese name: *fang-feng, feng-jou* 防風，防肉

Properties and actions: warm; acrid yet pleasant to taste. Antipyretic, analgesic, diaphoretic.

Indications: gout, colds, chills, headache, vertigo, general discomfort

Smilax
(Glabrous Greenbrier)

Botanical name: *Smilax glabra* (Liliaceae)
Pharmaceutical name: Rhizoma Smilacis—dried tubers
Chinese name: *tu-fu-ling* 土茯苓
From *Pen tsao kang mu*
Properties and actions: cool; bland. Diuretic, antispasmodic, antitoxic.
Indications: skin disorders, syphilis, stomatitis, indigestion, diarrhea, nephritis, cystitis, rheumatoid arthritis

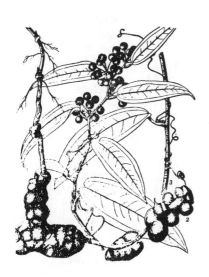

Smilax glabra

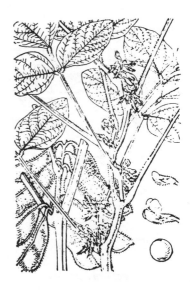

Glycine max

Soja

Botanical name: *Glycine max* (Leguminosae)
Pharmaceutical name: Semen Sojae Preparatum
Chinese name: *tan-tou-shih* 淡豆豉
From *Ming i pieh lu* (general drug)
Properties and actions: chilling properties, bitter to taste. Relaxes muscles, promotes perspiration, clears fever, and eliminates apprehension.
Indications: colds, irritability, vexation, dyspepsia, enteritis, diarrhea, vomiting

247

Sophora Flower
(Chinese Yellowberry Pagoda Tree)

Botanical name: *Sophora japonica* (Leguminosae)
Pharmaceutical name: Flos Sophorae
Chinese name: *huai-hua* 槐花
From *Shen Nung's Herbal*
Constituents: rutin
Properties and actions: bland and bitter. A hemostatic and analgesic. Strengthens the blood vessels.
Indications: hemoptysis, nosebleed, melena, hemorrhoids, hemorrhage, bloody diarrhea, metrorrhagia

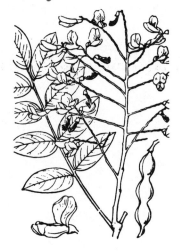

Sophora japonica

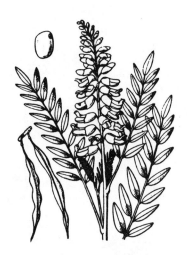

Sophora angustifolia

Sophora
(Shrubby Sophora)

Botanical name: *Sophora augustifolia, S. flavescens* (Leguminosae)
Pharmaceutical name: Radix Sophorae
Chinese name: *k'u-shen* 苦參
Constituents: sophoranol, matrine alkaloids, anagyrine, baptifoline, trifolirhizine, cytisine (sophorin)
Properties and actions: relieves fever, absorbs moisture, kills insects
Indications: dysentery, rectal bleeding, jaundice, tabes mesenterica, hematuria, scabies, hives

Stemona

Botanical name: *Stemona japonica, S. tuberosa* (Stemonaceae)
Pharmaceutical name: Radix Stemonae
Chinese name: *pai-pu* 百部
Constituents: stemonine
Properties and actions: slightly warm; sweetish, bitter taste. An anthelmintic and insecticide. Calms the respiratory center.
Indications: colds, coughs, phthisis, scabies

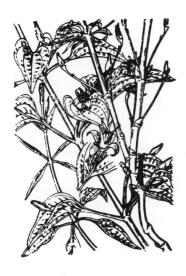

Stemona japonica

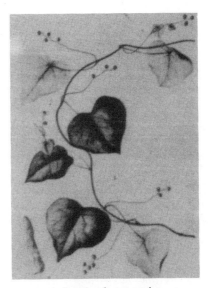

Stephania tetrandra

Stephania

Botanical name: *Stephania tetrandra* (Menispermaceae)
Pharmaceutical name: Radix Stephaniae
Chinese name: *fang-chi* 防己
Constituents: alkaloids, tetrandrine, tuduranine, sinomenine
Properties and actions: cool; bitter. Slightly poisonous. Diuretic, purgative, antispasmodic, antipyretic
Indications: edema, beriberi, spasms, pain in the arms and legs
Remarks: the botanical determination remains uncertain; the Chinese name is applied to several plants of the Menispermaceae family and the Aristolochia family.

Strychnine Tree (Nux-vomica)

Botanical name: *Strychnos nux-vomica* (Loganiaceae)

Pharmaceutical name: Semen Strychni

Chinese name: *fan-mu-pieh* 番木鼈

Constituents: fatty matter, glycoside, longanin, chlorogenic acid, mannosan, galactan, copper, the alkaloids strychnine and brucine

Properties and actions: cold; bitter. Spinal stimulant, bitter tonic.

Indications: debility with loss of appetite, convalescence from severe illness, acute diseases

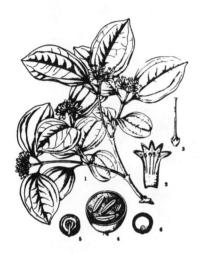

Strychnos nux-vomica

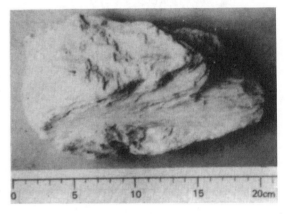

Talcum

Talc
(Soapstone)

Pharmaceutical name: Talcum

Chinese name: *hua-shih* 滑石

From *Shen Nung's Herbal*

Constituents: main chemical component is aqueous aluminum silicate, $Al_2O_3 \cdot 2\text{-}SiO_2 \cdot 2H_2O$.

Properties and actions: cold. Anti-inflammative. Cools, quenches thirst, renders diuresis.

Indications: urinary disorders, edema, dysuria, summer diarrhea, febrile dysentery, thirst, sunstroke

Tangerine (Citrus)

Botanical name: *Citrus chachiensis, C. tangerina, C. erythorosa, C. reticulata* (Rutaceae)

Pharmaceutical name: Pericarpium Citri Reticulatae

Chinese name: *ch'en-p'i* 陳皮

Constituents: isohesperidin, hesperic acid, protein, sugar

Properties and actions: warm; bitter and acrid. Antitussive, expectorant, tonic.

Indications: loss of vigor, leukorrhea, sputum, thoracic and abdominal distention, vomiting, diarrhea, cough

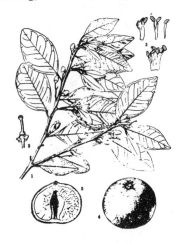

Citrus tangerina

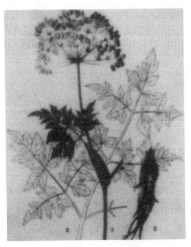

Angelica sinensis

Tang-kuei
(Chinese Angelica)

Botanical name: *Angelica sinensis* (Umbelliferae)

Pharmaceutical name: Radix Angelicae Sinensis

Chinese name: *tang-kuei* 當歸

Constituents: essential oil, resin, lactone, ligusticumic acid, *n*-dedecanol, butylphthalide

Properties and actions: warm; acrid, bitter. Hematinic, mild carminative. Stimulates circulation.

Indications: headache, lower back pain, cardiac and abdominal pain, dry stools, menstrual disorders, rheumatism, boils and ulcers, anemia, meridian and passageway obstructions

Terminalia
(Myrobalans)

Botanical name: *Terminalia chebula* (Combretaceae)
Pharmaceutical name: Fructus Chebulae
Chinese name: *ho-tzu* 訶子
From *Tang pen tsao*
Constituents: chebulic acid, fatty oil, tannin, ellagic acid
Properties and actions: warm; bitter, sour, and peppery. Astringent, expectorant, antitussive. Stimulates intestines, strengthens lungs.
Indications: chronic cough and hoarseness, chronic diarrhea and dysentery, prolapse of rectum, intestinal flatus and bloody stools, metrorrhagia and leukorrhea, seminal emission and excessive sweating

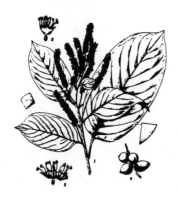

Terminalia chebula var. *grangetica*

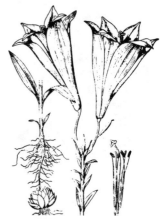

Lilium brownii var. *colchesteri*

Tiger Lily

Botanical name: *Lilium brownii* var. *colchesteri*, *L. tenuifolium*, *L. concolor* (Liliaceae)
Pharmaceutical name: Bulbus Lilii
Chinese name: *pai-ho* 百合
From *Shen Nung's Herbal* (general drug)
Constituents: starch, protein, fat, colchicein
Properties and actions: cold; bitter. Nutritive, antitussive, antipyretic, diuretic. Moistens lungs, clears fever, calms nerves.
Indications: hemoptysis, palpitations due to fear, edema, dysuria, weakness from coughing

Tokoro

Botanical name: *Dioscorea tokoro, D. sativa* (Dioscoreaceae)
Pharmaceutical name: Rhizoma Dioscoreae Bishie
Chinese name: *pi-hsieh* 草薢
From *Ming i pieh lu* (general drug)
Constituents: dioscin, dioscoreasapotoxin.
Properties and actions: bitter and bland. Antirheumatic, diuretic, and antidotal.
Indications: proteinuria, paralysis of lumbus and knees, noxious sores

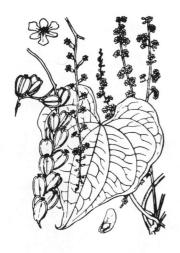

Dioscorea tokoro

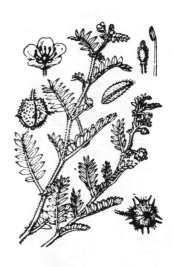

Tribulus terrestris

Tribulus
(Calthrop)

Botanical name: *Tribulus terrestris* (Zygophyllaceae)
Pharmaceutical name: Fructus Tribuli
Chinese name: *chi-li-tzu* 蒺藜子

Constituents: fixed oil, linoleic acid, an essential oil, tannin, phylloerythrin, vitamin A, a glycoside, phlobaphenes, peroxidase
Properties and actions: warm; bitter and pungent. A tonic. Promotes milk production in nursing mothers.
Indications: headaches, ophthalmia, eye disorders

Trichosanthes
(Snake Gourd)

Botanical name: *Trichosanthes kirilowii, T. multiloba* (Cucurbitaceae)
Pharmaceutical name: Semen et Radix Trichosanthis
Chinese name: *kua-lou, kua-lou-ken* 栝樓；栝樓根
Constituents: fatty oil
Properties and actions: cold, pleasant yet bitter to taste. Stabilizes pulmonary and intestinal functions, clears fevers, detoxifies, promotes salivation, aids pus drainage, reduces swelling.
Indications: sputum fever, cough, constipation, breast abscess, jaundice, difficult urination, bronchitis, laryngitis, mumps

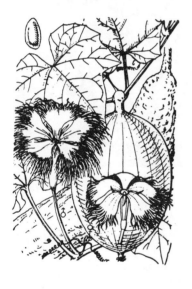

Trichosanthes kirilowii var. *japonica*

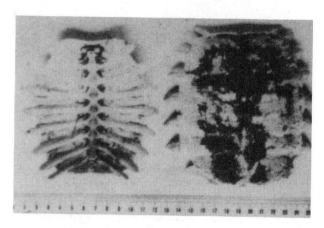

Carapax Amydae

Turtle Shell

Scientific name: *Amyda sinensis* (Triongchidae)
Pharmaceutical name: Carapax Amydae
Chinese name: *pieh-chia* 鼈甲
Properties and actions: nutritive, tonic. Cools fever.
Indications: debilitating fever, hardness and pain beneath the armpits, pain at the waist, amenorrhea, infantile epilepsy

Vitex

Botanical name: *Vitex rotundifolia* (Verbenaceae)

Pharmaceutical name: Fructus Viticis

Chinese name: *man-chin-tzu* 蔓荆子

From *Shen Nung's Herbal* (superior drug)

Constituents: camphene, vitexcarpin

Properties and actions: cool. Antipyretic, tonic.

Indications: headache, vertigo, eye disorders, convulsions, moist spasms

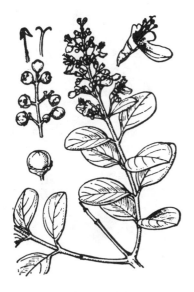
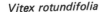

Vitex rotundifolia

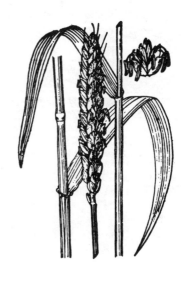

Triticum aestivum

Wheat

Botanical name: *Triticum sativum* (Gramineae)

Pharmaceutical name: Fructus Tritici Levis

Chinese name: *hsiao-mai* 小麥

From *Pen tsao kang mu*

Constituents: kernel contains large amounts of protein and carbohydrates

Properties and actions: reduces fevers

Indications: ephidrosis, night sweats, debilitating fever

Woodberry (Rubus)

Botanical name: *Rubus palmatus* (Rosaceae)
Pharmaceutical name: Fructus Rubi—dried unripe fruit
Chinese name: *fu-pen-tzu* 覆盆子
From *Ming-i-pieh-lu* (superior drug)
Properties and actions: warm; sweet, sour. Benefits respiration, imparts vigor, prevents graying.
Indications: impotence, spermatorrhea, enuresis

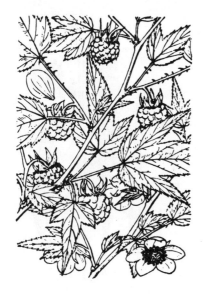

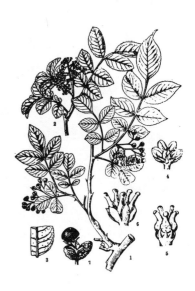

Rubus palmatus   *Zanthoxylum bungeanum*

Zanthoxylum
(Pepper Creeper)

Botanical name: *Zanthoxylum bungei* (Rutaceae)
Pharmaceutical name: Fructus Zanthoxyli Bungeani
Chinese name: *chuan-chiao* 川椒
Properties and actions: warm; pungent. Poisonous. Carminative, stimulant, sudorific, emmenagogue, astringent, anthelmintic. Warms the central organs, dispels chills and cold, counteracts moisture.
Indications: chilling pain, vomiting, diarrhea, worms

Zedoary

Botanical name: *Curcuma zedoaria* (Zingiberaceae)

Pharmaceutical name: Rhizoma Zedoariae

Chinese name: *o-shu* 莪蒁

Constituents: resin, essential oil, camphen, cineol, borneol, camphor, curcumin, zedoarin, gum, starch, zingiberen

Properties and actions: warm; bitter and pungent. Carminative, stomachic, peptic. Stimulates menstrual flow, promotes the flow of bile.

Indications: stagnancy of *ch'i* and blood, swelling pain in the heart and abdomen, food stagnancy, prolonged menstruation, contusions

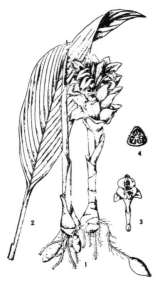

Curcuma zedoaria

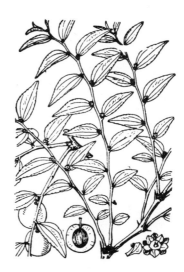

Zizyphus jujuba

Zizyphus

Botanical name: *Zizyphus jujuba* var. *spinosa* (Rhamnaceae)

Pharmaceutical name: Semen Zizyphi Spinosae

Chinese name: *suan-tsao-jen* 酸棗仁

From *Shen Nung's Herbal* (superior drug)

Constituents: betulin and betulinic acid.

Properties and actions: neutral, sour to taste. Nutritive tonic, sedative, and stomachic.

Indications: insomnia due to stress, palpitations due to anxiety, amnesia, thirst, weakness, ephidrosis

257

Herb Index

Chinese to English

Botanical/Scientific Name

Pharmaceutical Name

Formula Index

English to Chinese

275

Chinese to English

Formula Index

Books Listed in the Text

Chi chu nei ching (Commentary on the Yellow Emperor's Classic of Internal Medicine). Wang Ping. p. 9

Chien chin i fang (Precious Supplementary Prescriptions). Sun Su-miao (Sun Chen-jen). p. 8

Chien chin yao fang (Precious Prescriptions for Emergencies). Sun Su-miao (Sun Chen-jen). p. 8

Chin kuei yao lueh (Summaries of Household Remedies). Chang Chung-ching. pp. 6, 7, 59

Chu ping yuan hou lun (On Symptoms and Causes of Diseases). Chao Yuan-fang. p. 8

"The Historical Records of the Former Chin Dynasty", *Chinese Medical History*, December, 1953. Wang Fan. p. 1

Hsin hsiu pen ts'ao (New Revision of the Book of Herbs). Su Ching. p. 8

Huang ti nei ching. See *Nei ching.*

Mai ching (Book on Pulses). Wang Shu-ho. p. 27

Ming i pieh lu (Records of Famous Physicians). p. 7

Nan ching (Difficult Passages). Pien Chueh p. 27

Nei ching (The Yellow Emperor's Classic of Internal Medicine). Also *Huang ti nei ching.* pp. 3, 4, 14, 27, 43, 59, 66, 71, 72

Nei ching tai shu (Comments on the Yellow Emperor's Classic). Yang Shang-shan. p. 3

Pen ts'ao kang mu (General Catalog of Herbs). Li Shih-chen. p. 11

Pen ts'ao shih i (Supplement to the Book of Herbs). Chen Tsang-chi. pp. 8, 12

Shan hai ching (Book of the Mountain and the Sea). p. 5

Shang han lun (Treatise on Febrile Diseases). Chang Chung-ching. pp. 6, 9, 14, 43, 72

Shen nung pen ts'ao ching (Shen Nung's Book of Herbs). pp. 2, 7

Shih liao pen ts'ao (Dietetic Therapy of Herbs). Meng Hsien. Renamed by Chang Ting; originally called *Pu yao fang* or *Pi hsiao fang.* p. 9

Wai tai mi yao (Extra Medical Secrets). Wang Tao. p. 9

Yu hsueh chen chiu tu ching (Drawings and Discussions of Acupuncture and Moxibustion Points on the Bronze Man). Wang Wei-i. p. 9

Index

Index

Asthma, bronchial or childhood. See Respiratory system, diseases of
Astringents, 69, 76–7
Athlete's foot. See Skin diseases
Attacking and supplementing, 51–2

Back pain. See Chest or back pain
Baldness. See Skin diseases
Balms. See External medicines
Beriberi, postpartum. See Obstetrical problems
Bleeding. See Blood diseases, Obstetrical problems
ocular. See Ophthalmology
Blood
agents, 69
and *ch'i*, fire-purging formulas for, 75–6
disease, 44, 50, 55–6, 92–3
extravasated, 16, 40, 45, 48, 55, 59, 62
fire-purging formulas for, 75–6
formulas, 74
water, and *ch'i* theory of disease, 15–17, 50–1
Bone carvings, 1
Bone ulcer. See Surgery
Books
on drugs, 2, 5, 7–12
written during the Ching dynasty, 12
written during the Sung dynasty, 9, 10
Bowel movements in diagnosis, 23–4
Bronchial asthma. See Respiratory system, diseases of
Bronchial dilation. See Respiratory system, diseases of
Bronchitis. See Respiratory system, diseases of
Bronze man, 9
Burns. See Surgery

Carbuncle and dermatosis formulas, 77
Cardiac hyperfunction. See Palpitations and cardiac hyperfunction
Caries. See Dental problems
Carminatives, 74
Carved bone or *chia-ku-wen,* 1
Cataract. See Ophthalmology
Chang Ching-yueh
classification of formulas, 72
Chang Chung-ching, 6–9, 28
Chang Ting, 9
Chang Tzu-ho, 10
Chao Yuan-fang, 8
Chen En-fang, 10
Chen Shih-wen, 10

Chen Tsang-chi, 8
classification of formulas, 72
Chen Tzu-ming, 9
Chen Weng-chung, 9
Chest
or back pain, 118–120
distress and distention in diagnosis, 37
pain in diagnosis, 24–5
Chia-ku-wen (bone carvings), 1
Ch'i
ascending, 16
and blood, fire-purging formulas for, 76–6
blood and water theory of disease, 15–7, 50–1
disease, 44, 50, 55–9, 62–3, 76, 109
fire-purging formulas for, 75–6
formulas, 73–4
melancholic, 16–7
mobile, 16–7
stagnant, 29, 31
still, 16–7
Chi-chun, Wu, 12
Chien I, 9
Chien, Tsou, 4
Childbirth fever. See Obstetrical problems
Chill-dispelling formulas, 74
Chills, 21, 47, 47, 57, 61, 66, 68, 122–3
Ching dynasty, books written during, 12
Ching, Su, 8
Chi, Tung, 9
Cholecystitis. See Digestive system, diseases of
Cholelithiasis. See Digestive system, diseases of
Chou li tien kuan system, 4
Chronic constipation, 63
Chu Tan-hsi, 10
Chueh, Pien, 27
Chung-ching, Chang, 6–9
Circulation in diagnosis
Circulatory system, diseases of, 30, 86–9
Cirrhosis of the liver. See Digestive system, diseases of
Cold agents, 68
Cold, common. See Respiratory system, diseases of
Color
of drugs, 65
of skin in diagnosis, 20
of tongue in diagnosis, 44
Conformation, 19, 51, 72–3
external and internal wind, 74
inside and outside, 52
Congenital anomalies. See Gynecological problems
Congestion and hardness in lower abdomen, 40

304

Index

Index

Index

Umbilicus
in diagnosis, 36
numbness below, 40
Urination in diagnosis, 24
Urticaria. See Skin diseases
Uterus
prolapse of. See Gynecological problems
retroversion of. See Gynecological problems
swelling of. See Gynecological problems

Vermiculation, intestinal, 41
Vesicles. See Pediatrics, Skin diseases
Vicarious menstruation. See Gynecological
problems
Vision-improving formulas, 77
Vomiting, 121. See also Nausea
in diagnosis, 24
method, 48

Wang An, 12
Wang Fan, 1
Wang Ping, 9
Wang Shu-ho, 27
Wang Tao, 9
Wang Wei-i, 9
Wan-su, Liu, 10

Warmers (upper, middle and lower), 27, 39, 58
Warming method, 49
contraindications for, 49
and removing, 51
Warts. See Skin diseases
Water
accumulation, 56
blood and *ch'i* theory of disease, 15–7, 50–1
disease, 48, 109–111
Weak and strong, 14, 51
Wei-i, Wang, 9
Weng-chung, Chen, 9
Whooping cough. See Respiratory system, dis-
eases of
Wind
conformation, external and internal, 74
and moisture disease. See Rheumatism
Wu Chi-chun, 12
Wu I-lo, 12

Yang Shang-shan, 3
Yang and yin *ch'i,* 16, 49, 57
Yin and yang, 14
ch'i, 16, 32, 43, 51
in disease, 6, 33, 50, 60
drugs to balance, 65–6
the six disease stages, 14, 45
Yuan-fang, Chao, 8